THE

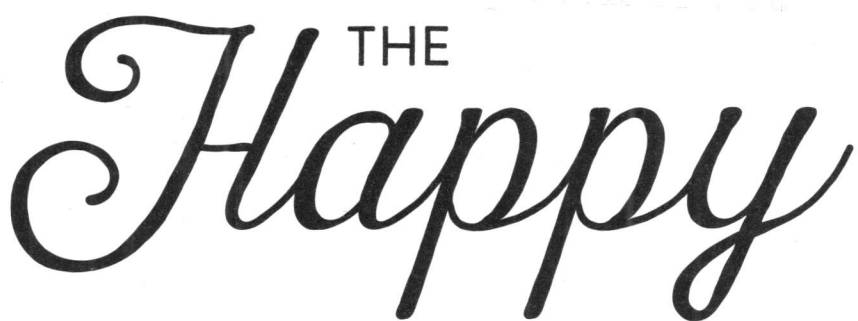
Happy

MENOPAUSE
GUIDE TO
ENERGY

Jackie Lynch

THE
Happy
MENOPAUSE
GUIDE TO
ENERGY

NUTRITION TO REJUVENATE
YOUR BRAIN & BODY

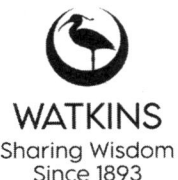

WATKINS
Sharing Wisdom
Since 1893

The Happy Menopause Guide to Energy
Jackie Lynch

This edition first published in the UK and USA in 2025 by
Watkins, an imprint of Watkins Media Limited
Unit 11, Shepperton House, 89-93 Shepperton Road
London, N1 3D
enquiries@watkinspublishing.com

1 2 3 4 5 6 7 8 9 10

Commissioning Editor: Fiona Robertson
Managing Editor: Daniel Culver
Production: Uzma Taj
Text design: Glen Wilkins

Typeset by JCS Publishing Ltd

Printed and bound by CPI Group (UK) Ltd, Croydon, CR0 4YY

The manufacturer's authorised representative in the EU for product safety is:
eucomply OÜ - Pärnu mnt 139b-14, 11317 Tallinn, Estonia,
hello@eucompliancepartner.com, www.eucompliancepartner.com

A CIP record for this book is available from the British Library

ISBN: 978-1-78678-967-9 (Paperback)
ISBN: 978-1-83681-014-8 (eBook)

www.watkinspublishing.com

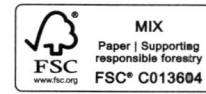

CONTENTS

For Mum & Dad, who always
encouraged and supported me
in every endeavour.

I know you'd both be tickled pink
to see me publish my fourth book.

INTRODUCTION
WELCOME TO MY ENERGY CLINIC

Are you tired of being tired? Do you wake up feeling exhausted before you've even begun your day? If so, you've come to the right place.

The Happy Menopause Guide to Energy offers a book version of my real-world nutrition clinic – a place where you'll learn how to reignite your energy, restore your vitality and feel like yourself again. Step by step, this book will guide you through The Happy Menopause Energy Clinic, to help you take charge of your wellbeing and create your personal Energy Action Plan. Let's get started!

Constant fatigue can be debilitating. When we're not producing the energy we need, life feels like an uphill battle. Tiredness affects every aspect of our lives:

- **Brain fog:** making it harder to think clearly or focus
- **Poor memory:** forgetting even the simplest things
- **Irritability:** feeling on edge for no apparent reason
- **Anxiety & low mood:** feeling uneasy or weighed down, with a lingering sense of dread or sadness
- **Weakness & exhaustion:** lacking the strength, stamina and resilience to deal with challenges or to do the things you love

In my menopause nutrition clinic, women consult me for a variety of reasons, but they all share one thing in common: they're exhausted. Often, they dismiss their tiredness as a natural consequence of ageing or an inevitable side-effect of menopause. And, like so many women, they soldier on, pushing through the exhaustion because that's what women do.

But it doesn't have to be that way.

This book is here to show you how to feel energized, positive and productive every day. By understanding the root causes of fatigue and taking simple, practical actions to address them, you can put the spring back in your step.

When you reclaim your energy, you'll rediscover joy, creativity and the ability to thrive in your everyday life.

A brief overview of menopause

It might help to think of menopause as the reverse of puberty: a major transition for the body that doesn't happen overnight. During puberty, your body starts producing more oestrogen and progesterone, and your periods mark the beginning of your fertile years. As you approach menopause, these hormones start to fluctuate significantly, which can trigger a variety of symptoms. Over time, levels will decline, the ovaries stop producing oestrogen, and your periods come to an end.

There's often confusion around the terms "perimenopausal", "menopausal" and "post-menopausal", so let's clarify the differences and help you identify your stage.

Perimenopause	This pre-menopausal phase is when a whole range of symptoms can begin, from psychological and emotional changes to physical issues such as hot flushes and night sweats. In fact, there are over 35 common symptoms of perimenopause, which can affect women in various ways. The perimenopause may even start in your early 40s and can last for several years as hormonal changes gradually lead to menopause.
Menopause	While the term "menopause" is frequently used as shorthand for the entire transition — and I'll often do the same throughout this book — technically, it refers to just one day: the point at which it has been exactly 12 months since your last period. The average age of menopause in the UK and USA is 51, but this can vary widely, with some women experiencing it earlier or later.
Post-menopause	If you haven't had a period for 12 months, you're officially post-menopausal. Some symptoms may persist for a while, but your body will gradually adapt to its new hormonal balance, and many symptoms should diminish over time. However, oestrogen and progesterone do more than regulate your menstrual cycle – they also support bone density, heart health, muscle function and pelvic floor. As these hormone levels decline, it's important to pay attention to these areas of your health on a long-term basis.

No two women have the same experience of menopause. Around 20 per cent of women sail through with very few symptoms, while another 20 per cent have a much harder time, with severe or prolonged symptoms. Most of us fall somewhere in between, experiencing some but not all symptoms. These symptoms can come and go, and their severity can vary greatly.

It's important to arm yourself with the right information so you can make an informed decision about the best approach for you in managing your menopause, rather than being swayed by someone else's experience, which may be very different from your own. There is no one-size-fits-all solution – it's about what works best for you as an individual. So don't beat yourself up if you initially think you'll take a "natural" approach and then decide that the right choice is hormone replacement therapy (HRT, or MHT in the USA). It could be a gamechanger for you in terms of your symptoms, and might help your energy levels too.

Similarly, if you're feeling great and don't feel the need for HRT, that's perfectly fine too. Speak to your doctor or the practice nurse at your local surgery, and check out the back of this book for reliable and evidence-based resources to help you make the right decision for you.

While menopause can bring challenges, it's also a natural transition and an opportunity to prioritize your health and wellbeing. That's why I've created *The Happy Menopause* series of books and podcasts, which focus on empowering you to embrace this next phase of life with confidence.

The menopause & your energy levels

Are you blaming menopause for your lack of energy? That's perfectly understandable – there's certainly a connection. The hormonal fluctuations of perimenopause and menopause affect every system in the body, including those involved in energy production. So, it's no wonder you feel more tired than you used to.

However, it's important not to assume this is just how life will be from now on. Energy is a complex issue, and there are many other potential reasons why you might feel physically or mentally drained.

In this book, we'll explore how functional imbalances, nutrient deficiencies and lifestyle factors can affect your brain and body. Keep reading to discover how you can revitalize yourself.

HOW TO USE THIS BOOK

My previous book, *The Happy Menopause: Smart Nutrition to Help You Flourish*, is a symptom-by-symptom guide designed to help women navigate perimenopause, menopause and post-menopause by making clever nutritional choices. It also includes a dedicated chapter that delves into the hormonal changes of perimenopause and menopause, providing a deeper understanding of what's happening in your body, which you might find especially helpful. The book is designed as a flexible, modular resource that you can dip in and out of, addressing the issues most relevant to you.

The Happy Menopause Guide to Energy takes a different approach. This book is a deep dive into the science of energy production in the body, the impact of the menopause on your energy, and how your diet and lifestyle can help.

As a nutritionist, I've guided thousands of women in my clinic through the challenges of perimenopause and menopause, helping them feel strong, energized and positive. I launched my podcast, "The Happy Menopause", in 2019 to share expert advice with women who couldn't consult me directly. Since then, it's reached hundreds of thousands of listeners and has inspired me to create an online community: The Happy Menopause Club. This deeply rewarding experience has shown me the real-life impact of offering accessible, practical support.

The Happy Menopause Guide to Energy is the latest addition to the collection. It mirrors the approach I'd take with you in my nutrition clinic, guiding you through a 5-step personalized process to uncover your energy weak points. Each step in The Happy Menopause Energy Clinic builds on the last, helping you develop tailored strategies for renewed vitality and wellbeing.

To get the most out of the book, it's best to work through it systematically, step by step. Each section will guide you on your journey toward better energy and wellbeing and encourage you to reflect on what you've learned. You'll be using your findings to create your own personal Energy Action Plan when you reach the end of the book.

Here's exactly what you can expect as you journey through The Happy Menopause Energy Clinic:

- **Step 1: Understand the Science of Energy: Nutrition, Mitochondria & Menopause**

This chapter offers a straightforward look at how the body produces energy. I've always believed that understanding the "why" behind something is just as important as knowing the "what", especially when it comes to making changes in your life. When you grasp what the body needs to create energy, it becomes much easier to motivate yourself to make the dietary choices that support this process.

In my nutrition clinic, I make a point of explaining the reasoning behind every piece of advice I give. After all, we're adults, and you deserve to understand why you're receiving a particular recommendation. Armed with this knowledge, you can make informed, positive choices about your health. This part of the book lays the foundation for the next steps in your energy journey, giving you the understanding and confidence to move forward.

- **Step 2: Know Your Numbers: The Key Health Checks Every Woman Needs**

As we navigate perimenopause and menopause, it's crucial to take a proactive approach to routine health checks, even if you feel generally fit and well. Subtle imbalances could be draining your energy and might also signal potential health issues further down the line.

In this section, you'll discover the health checks you need to prioritize and how to interpret the results. With this understanding, you'll be better equipped to have meaningful discussions with your doctor about what the findings mean and how they can guide your next steps.

Using a notebook to log any action points will be important, as these will contribute to the personal Energy Action Plan that you'll make once you've worked your way through the next three chapters.

- **Step 3: Nutrition Essentials: Complete the 14-Day Energy Boost Programme**

Once you've explored the science and completed your key health checks, the next step is to investigate the essentials of good nutrition and to complete the 14-Day Energy Boost Programme. Often, simple changes to your diet can bring about a remarkable improvement in energy and overall wellbeing in just a short space of time. During an initial nutritional consultation in my real-world clinic, one of the first things I do is analyse a client's food diary to ensure they're getting the basics right.

In this section, we'll examine the role of macronutrients and optimal hydration in supporting your energy levels. Macronutrients – proteins, fats and carbohydrates – are nutrients you need in large amounts. Achieving the right balance is essential to power your brain and body, and this balance plays a key role in supporting you through perimenopause, menopause and beyond. We'll delve into each macronutrient, with lists of good food sources to help you optimize your diet and practical steps to take to implement the dietary changes. Throughout this section there will be plenty of opportunities to reflect on key takeaways and jot them down in your notebook as potential objectives for your Energy Action Plan.

Then it's time to begin your 14-Day Energy Boost Programme. I've carefully designed this plan to help you balance your macronutrients and hydration. You should start to notice improvements in energy, strength and stamina within days. It's important to complete this programme fully before moving on. While it may be tempting to skip ahead, finishing the 14 days first will ensure that any macronutrient imbalances are addressed. This will make the energy quizzes in the next section more accurate and reflective of your post-programme energy levels.

- ## Step 4: Discover Targeted Solutions for Micronutrient Imbalances

With the energy basics of your diet sorted, you should already be feeling the benefits. In this chapter we'll explore more complex factors that might be impacting your physical and mental energy, such as micronutrient (i.e. vitamin and mineral) deficiencies or functional imbalances.

In my real-world nutrition clinic, I'd often recommend blood tests at this stage. In this virtual energy clinic, you'll use a series of symptom quizzes instead. Your quiz scores will highlight specific energy weak points, and in some cases you may be advised to consult your doctor for blood tests to confirm any suspected deficiencies or imbalances. You'll also receive practical guidance on interpreting test results, giving you the information you need to make informed choices about next steps.

Each quiz result will include an explanation of potential issues, how they relate to menopause, and practical diet and lifestyle strategies to address them. This will include lists of foods rich in the relevant vitamins or minerals, with simple suggestions for prioritizing them in your diet. You'll also learn which supplements might benefit you and how to use them safely.

There's plenty of opportunity for reflection as you work through the advice in the book. Each section, from the end of Step 2 onwards, includes an "Easy Ways to ..." summary which features some helpful suggestions to get you started. The more you jot down in your notebook, the better equipped you'll be to create your personal Energy Action Plan at the end of your journey through The Happy Menopause Energy Clinic.

- **Step 5: Energy Gain or Energy Drain? Make Lifestyle Choices to Improve Your Vitality**

The final piece of the energy jigsaw puzzle is lifestyle. In the previous chapters, you will have learned how various factors work together to support your energy levels. Smart lifestyle choices are another integral part of the energy equation.

This section explores the elements that can influence your energy positively or negatively – or sometimes both! We'll be looking at caffeine, alcohol, sleep, exercise, stress and inflammation. You'll learn how each of these impacts your energy and menopause symptoms, along with strategies and advice to manage them effectively.

As you read, take note of the factors that resonate with you and reflect on practical steps you can take to make positive changes. All of this will contribute to your personal Energy Action Plan.

- **Bringing It All Together: Design Your Personal Energy Action Plan**

This is your moment! You've reached the end of your journey through The Happy Menopause Energy Clinic and it's time to put everything into practice. This section is all about you, and it's where your notebook truly comes into its own. The notes and reflections you've gathered while working through each chapter are your toolkit for success.

With the guidance provided here, and drawing on the insights that you've compiled, you'll create an Energy Action Plan that's tailored to your needs. It will help you restore both physical and mental energy, and ensure you can keep them thriving for the long term.

GETTING READY TO BEGIN

Before you dive in, I recommend treating yourself to a beautiful notebook. Choose one with a cover that inspires you and paper that feels wonderful. This notebook will be your trusted companion as you journey through The Happy Menopause Energy Clinic.

Set SMART energy objectives

At the end of each section, I'll encourage you to reflect on what you've learned and jot down the points that feel most important or relevant to you. This is essential, as you'll use these notes at the end of the book to create your personalized 5-step Energy Action Plan.

With each action point, you might find it helpful to think in terms of a SMART objective: Specific – Measurable – Achievable – Realistic – Timebound. This will ensure that you're setting yourself up for success and makes it more likely that you'll follow through on your goal.

For example, instead of saying, "I'm going to eat more protein", which is quite vague, try setting a goal like, "Starting tomorrow, I'll add 2 tablespoons of seeds to my morning cereal." It's clear, measurable and easily achievable.

Take your time

It's important to go at your own pace. In my clinic, a nutrition programme typically unfolds over 12–16 weeks. You don't need to rush; taking the time to absorb and implement what you've learned is the best way to ensure lasting success, especially if you're already feeling overloaded.

For example, Step 3 introduces a simple 14-day Energy Boost Programme designed to get the basics right and address any obvious imbalances. While it might be tempting to jump straight into the symptom quizzes in the next chapter, waiting is key. Completing the Energy Boost Programme first will give you a clearer picture of your energy levels and help you get more accurate results from the quizzes.

By taking it one step at a time, you'll be able to build on each section's learnings and fully empower yourself to take control of your energy and wellbeing. This thoughtful, measured approach is the best way to achieve long-term success, although you should already start to see improvements within just a few days of starting the 14-Day Energy Boost Programme.

Follow this roadmap to happiness & energy

I'm excited to share this journey with you. From my clinical experience, I've seen the transformative impact it can have when women in menopause rediscover their energy. It's not just about feeling less tired – it's about reclaiming your vitality, your productivity and your joy in everyday life.

This is your time for self-care, your moment to focus on *you*. Too often, your own health and wellbeing get pushed to the bottom of the list. But here, in The Happy Menopause Energy Clinic, you'll find a space dedicated entirely to your needs.

Through the practical and achievable solutions in this guide, I hope to help you restore your energy, enhance your wellbeing and embrace a healthy, happy menopause – and beyond.

I'm so pleased to see you in The Happy Menopause Energy Clinic. Let's get started!

Jackie

STEP 1

UNDERSTAND THE SCIENCE OF ENERGY: NUTRITION, MITOCHONDRIA & MENOPAUSE

When you're tired, everything requires more effort, and it can all seem so difficult! It's tough to motivate yourself to get up in the morning or to get off the sofa when your very bones seem weary. Creative thinking, memory, concentration and motivation go out of the window; worry and dread can creep in; and your stores of patience often disappear along with your energy. When fatigue sets in, it can be very hard to carry out all the different daily tasks and obligations with a smile, and the idea of actually enjoying life may seem pretty distant.

Why is this? Tiredness has a broad impact on both the brain and the body because every single cell requires energy to function. To understand how we can support our energy levels and banish fatigue, we need to look at how the body produces energy. This will help us identify what we can do to facilitate that process. By understanding what our body needs to perform at its best, it becomes easier to commit to the necessary diet and lifestyle changes.

We're now taking the first step on your journey through The Happy Menopause Energy Clinic – learning about the "why" that will help motivate you to stick with the changes I'm going to suggest. I'll keep things as simple and straightforward as I would when discussing the process with my real-world clients, so read on for a short explanation of how energy works.

THE SCIENCE OF ENERGY: HOW YOUR BODY POWERS YOU

Let's dive into the amazing process your body uses to turn food into the fuel you need to live, think and move.

How it works: the big picture

1. **The raw materials of energy**

   Everything starts with the food you eat. Your body breaks it down into smaller, useful pieces which act as your fuel:

   o **Carbohydrates** become glucose (your body's favourite quick-energy source).

   o **Fats** are turned into fatty acids (great for longer-lasting energy).

   o **Proteins** break down into amino acids, which are vital for building and repairing your body, and can also help with energy when needed.

   These three macronutrients – carbohydrates, fats and proteins – are the raw materials your body needs to create energy.

2. **Meet your energy factories**

   Inside every cell of your body, there are lots of tiny, hardworking rod-shaped structures called mitochondria. These little factories are where the magic happens – they turn the food you eat into energy. Respiration is the fancy term for this process, but don't confuse it with breathing, which is technically called ventilation. You'll hear a lot more about mitochondria as we go through the book.

3. **The star of the show: ATP**
   The energy created in your mitochondria is stored in molecules called adenosine triphosphate (ATP). Think of ATP as your body's rechargeable batteries. These little energy units power *everything*, from moving your muscles to firing up your brain.

A simple chain reaction: turning food into energy

You might remember learning about energy production in high school chemistry, a process known as the citric acid or Krebs cycle. Here's how it all comes together:

- Your body breaks down the food you eat into glucose, fatty acids and amino acids, which will be your fuel.
- These fuel molecules enter your cells and head to the mitochondria, which get to work.
- Inside the mitochondria, the fuel molecules meet oxygen and create ATP, those wonderful little energy storage units. (See the Appendix for a step-by-step breakdown of the process.)
- ATP is now ready to fuel your body whenever and wherever you need it – from getting out of bed to chasing after the bus!

For now, just remember **food + oxygen = energy,** *thanks to your mitochondria and their trusty ATP batteries!*

THE ROLE OF NUTRIENTS IN ENERGY PRODUCTION

Your body needs a combination of macronutrients (i.e. carbohydrates, fats and proteins, which act as your fuel) and micronutrients (i.e. vitamins and minerals that support the energy production process) to keep your engine running smoothly.

Macronutrients: the big three

1. **Carbohydrates: your body's favourite fuel**
   Carbohydrates are quick and efficient. They're rapidly broken down into glucose, which is your body's main energy source.

2. **Fats: long-lasting energy**
   Fat is like a slow-burning candle, providing a steady energy supply for lower-intensity activities or when carbohydrates run low.

3. **Proteins: more than just a backup**
   Protein plays a crucial role in building and repairing your body, from muscles to tissues. While it's not your body's first choice for energy, it's there to help when needed. Amino acids from protein can be converted into glucose if your body runs low on other fuels. It's very important to eat enough protein to support your overall health, energy and strength.

Micronutrients: the essential helpers

These don't provide energy directly but are crucial for keeping the whole energy production process running smoothly:

- **B vitamins (B1, B2, B3, B5, B6, B9 (folate) and B12):** These act as spark plugs for your body, helping every stage of energy production. They also assist in the production of red blood cells, ensuring oxygen reaches your cells.
- **Iron:** Think of iron as the oxygen delivery driver. It's vital for transporting oxygen in your blood, which your mitochondria need to make energy.
- **Magnesium:** This multitasker mineral activates ATP and supports nearly every chemical reaction in energy production.
- **Co-enzyme Q10 (CoQ10):** found in your mitochondria, CoQ10 helps produce ATP efficiently. It is mostly produced directly by the body, although it is found in small amounts in some foods, including oily fish, nuts and seeds.
- **Antioxidants (vitamins A, C and E):** these protect your mitochondria from damage caused by the wear and tear of energy production, keeping everything running smoothly.

By understanding how these nutrients work together, you'll have the tools to keep your body energized and running at its best. We'll keep exploring the process throughout the book, so you can feel confident in nourishing your amazing, energy-producing machine.

THE MIGHTY MITOCHONDRIA

Let's zoom in on your body's energy factories, the mitochondria.

These tiny structures pack a big punch, producing about 90 per cent of the energy your body needs. Without them, you wouldn't be able to think, move or thrive, so it's important to nurture them.

The number of mitochondria in each cell depends on how much energy that cell needs. Each individual muscle, brain and liver cell can contain thousands of mitochondria, all working away tirelessly keep you going.

What makes mitochondria special?

Mitochondria aren't just energy producers – they're surprisingly clever! They have their own DNA, separate from the DNA in the nucleus of your cells that determines things like your eye colour or height. This mitochondrial DNA (or mtDNA) helps your mitochondria produce energy and keep your cells healthy.

But here's the catch: mtDNA is more delicate than the DNA in your cell's nucleus. It doesn't repair itself as easily, so it's more vulnerable to damage from things like oxidative stress (a by-product of energy production), nutrient deficiencies, toxins and even ageing. This damage can lead to reduced energy and has been linked to conditions like Alzheimer's and Parkinson's disease.

To protect your mtDNA, it's important to give your mitochondria plenty of support, by eating a diet rich in antioxidant vitamins (A, C and E), which act as a shield against oxidative stress. You'll learn how to prioritize these key vitamins as you progress through the book.

A Mother's Gift

We inherit our mitochondrial DNA from our mother. She passes it on to both her sons and daughters, but only the daughters will be able to pass it on to their children.

Mitochondria & menopause

During perimenopause and menopause, falling oestrogen levels can take a toll on your mitochondria. That's one reason why you might feel like your energy levels have dipped or your brain isn't working as sharply as it used to.

Oestrogen helps mitochondria in several ways:
- **Energy production:** It helps regulate the production of ATP (your energy storage molecules), so a reduction in oestrogen can impact your ability to store energy effectively.
- **Antioxidant protection:** Oestrogen shields mtDNA from the damaging impact of oxidative stress, so when levels drop your mitochondria are left more vulnerable.
- **Mitochondrial growth:** Oestrogen supports the creation of new mitochondria, so fewer mitochondria are made as levels decline.

This all contributes to the physical and mental changes many women experience during menopause.

But the good news is, there's a lot you can do to support your mitochondria and reclaim your energy!

Supporting your mitochondria

Your diet and lifestyle choices play a powerful role in keeping your mitochondria healthy. These are some of the ways you can nurture your mitochondria – we'll explore them in more detail in the rest of the book:
- **Eat a balanced diet** rich in nutrients, including antioxidants.
- **Maintain steady blood sugar levels** by avoiding spikes and crashes.
- **Get regular exercise**, but avoid overdoing it, which can strain your mitochondria.

- **Prioritize quality sleep**, as your body repairs itself while you rest.
- **Manage stress**, since chronic stress can harm your energy production.
- **Stay hydrated**, as even mild dehydration can affect energy levels.
- **Limit toxin exposure** by avoiding foods containing artificial additives and reducing contact with pollutants.

WHAT'S NEXT?

I hope Step 1 of your journey has helped you understand just how incredible – and important – your mitochondria are. They're the powerhouse behind your energy and wellbeing, and by taking care of them, you're investing in a vibrant, fulfilling life.

In the chapters ahead, we'll move from the science to the practical. As you progress through The Happy Menopause Energy Clinic, you'll learn how to make small, manageable changes that will have a big impact on your mitochondrial function and your energy. Ready to take action?

As a first step, why don't you start using your notebook? Take a moment to jot down anything from this section that resonated with you. Reflecting now will help you get the most out of what's to come.

A few simple questions to guide your thoughts

1. Was there anything about this breakdown of how energy is produced in the body that stood out to you?
2. How do you feel about making changes to support your energy levels?
3. How do you plan to support your mitochondria, going forward?

STEP 2

KNOW YOUR NUMBERS: THE KEY HEALTH CHECKS EVERY WOMAN NEEDS

It's important to take a proactive approach to your health and to make sure that you're on top of the medical side of things. For example, when did you last have your blood pressure, your blood glucose or your cholesterol checked? In my real-world clinic, these are details I would ask for in the pre-consultation health questionnaire, because imbalances in any of these areas may be linked to your tiredness. Do you know what's normal for you?

It's easy to let things slide if you feel generally fit and well, but as you move through the menopause, it's important to keep on top of these matters.

The work you put into supporting your health now will lay the groundwork for you to be fit and well in later life.

Should I see my doctor about my lack of energy?

Underlying health issues can contribute to tiredness. If you start to experience unusually low energy, or if your fatigue is persistent and unrelieved by rest, your first port of call should always be your doctor.

They will want to run a number of tests to rule out any medical condition or potential imbalances that could be contributing to your symptoms. Areas they will explore as a priority would include diabetes, cholesterol and blood pressure. They may also investigate thyroid function and certain nutrient deficiencies, such as a vitamin B12, folate, iron or vitamin D.

Prior to the menopause, the risk of coronary heart disease is much lower for women than for men. Post-menopause this changes, with the loss of the protective effects of oestrogen on the heart muscle, and the risk for women becomes the same as for men. There is also a greater propensity to issues with high cholesterol or diabetes once you've transitioned through the menopause.

This is why it's so important to know your numbers and what is standard for you.

UNDERSTANDING YOUR TEST RESULTS

Your doctor will explain your results to you and let you know what action may be required, but here are some simple guidelines and reference ranges which you might find helpful.

1. **Diabetes**

   If your doctor wants to rule out an issue with diabetes, they may test either fasting blood glucose levels or HbA1C, which is glycated haemoglobin.

   Blood glucose

   A blood glucose test is usually taken after fasting overnight and before eating breakfast, which is when the blood sugar should be at its lowest. This provides a snapshot of the glucose status at that specific time.

   Blood glucose is usually measured in millimoles per litre (mmol/L) or milligrams per decilitre (mg/dL). The reference ranges for a fasting blood glucose test are:

   Normal: 4–5.4mmol/L or 72–99mg/dL

   Prediabetes: 5.5–6.9mmol/L or 100–125mg/dL

   Diabetes: >7mmol/L or >126mg/dL

HbA1C

HbA1C measures the amount of sugar that is bound to the haemoglobin in a red blood cell. This will provide an on-going average of blood sugar levels, because the lifespan of a red blood cell is three months. This is likely to provide a more effective reflection of your blood glucose status.

HbA1C is measured in millimoles per mole (mmol/mol) or sometimes as a percentage. These are the standard reference ranges.

Normal: <42mmol/mol or <6%

Prediabetes: 42–47mmol/mol or 6–6.4%

Diabetes: >48mmol/mol or >6.5%

2. Blood pressure

Your blood pressure is measured with two numbers; for example, a reading might be 120/80mmHg. The higher number is the systolic pressure, which is when your heart pumps and the pressure is at its highest. The lower number is the diastolic pressure, which is when your heart is at rest and the pressure is at its lowest.

A normal reading is considered to be between 90–120mmHg for the systolic (higher) number and 60–80mmHg for the diastolic (lower) number.

3. **Cholesterol**

Cholesterol is a waxy fat-like substance which is found in every cell of our body. About 80 per cent of our cholesterol is produced in the liver, although it is present in animal products such as red meat, shellfish, dairy and eggs.

It generally has a pretty bad press, but cholesterol is actually the stuff of life. We need it to build cells and it is used by the body to produce sex hormones. It's required for the synthesis of vitamin D, and for the production of bile, to support our digestion. It's also important for the brain and nervous system.

You can see that cholesterol itself isn't bad for us. However, imbalances of cholesterol can be problematic and may increase the risk of cardiovascular disease.

Cholesterol is transported around the body by carrier proteins called low-density lipoprotein (LDL) and high-density lipoprotein (HDL). LDL carries the cholesterol to the cells and tissues, and HDL carries it away to the liver where it is broken down and sent off for excretion from the body.

The correct balance of LDL and HDL are very important to reduce the risk of cholesterol building up in the arteries.

Excessive levels of triglycerides are also a potential risk factor for cardiovascular disease. This is another fatty substance that circulates in the blood. Triglycerides store unused calories and can be used as a source of energy. However, high levels can contribute to hardening of the arteries.

Oestrogen & cholesterol

Oestrogen supports fat metabolism in the liver, so the drop in oestrogen during perimenopause and menopause can affect your HDL–LDL balance and may increase levels of triglycerides. This is why you need to keep an eye on cholesterol levels during and post-menopause.

You're unlikely to experience obvious symptoms from high cholesterol or triglycerides, so a regular blood test is important to assess your levels and to ensure that your diet and lifestyle are helping you maintain the correct balance.

Here are the recommended reference ranges for a standard cholesterol test for women in the UK (measured in millimoles per litre) and the USA (measured in milligrams per decilitre).

Cholesterol type	UK (mmol/L)	USA (mg/dL)
Total cholesterol	4.1–5.0mmol/L	125–200mg/dL
HDL	1.2–2.3mmol/L	50–80mg/dL
LDL	1.2–3.0mm/L	50–100mg/dL
Non-HDL	<4.0mmol/L	<130mg/dL
Triglycerides	<1.7mmol/L	<150mg/dL

WHAT TO DO NEXT

1. If you haven't had your blood pressure, blood glucose or cholesterol checked in the past two years, book an appointment with your doctor today. In the UK these tests are available free on the NHS once you're over 40, but it's important to take the initiative and book yourself in – after all, it's easy to be overlooked if you don't ask.

2. If you've had these tests recently but haven't seen the results, contact your surgery for a copy to understand your current status.

3. Record all your results for future reference to help you stay on track. Aim to schedule routine checks every couple of years to manage your health proactively.

4. If you're worried about your blood pressure, consider using a simple blood pressure monitor, which you can buy online at a reasonable cost. If your readings are higher at the clinic due to anxiety (known as "white coat syndrome"), your doctor might suggest wearing a home monitor for 24 hours to get a more accurate reading.

Easy ways to balance blood glucose and promote heart health

- **Get the balance right**: Ensure your diet includes the correct proportions of proteins, fats and carbohydrates. (See page 113 for detailed advice on blood sugar balance.)
- **Eat a rainbow**: Include a variety of brightly coloured vegetables in your meals throughout the week to benefit from heart-healthy antioxidants.

- **Enjoy berries for your heart**: Berries are packed with polyphenols, plant compounds that help lower the risk of cardiovascular disease. Eat them regularly.
- **Opt for oats**: Rich in beta-glucans, oats support healthy cholesterol levels.
- **Fish for health**: Include oily fish, such as mackerel, salmon or sardines, in your diet three times a week. They're rich in omega-3, which supports a healthy blood pressure.
- **Be mindful of saturated fats**: Moderate your intake of foods such as cheese, butter and red meat to help regulate LDL cholesterol levels.
- **Cut back on sugar**: Avoid sugary snacks, baked goods and sweet drinks to manage blood sugar levels and reduce the risk of triglyceride build-up.
- **Drink alcohol in moderation**: Support a healthy blood pressure by keeping your alcohol consumption within recommended guidelines (see page 226).
- **Stay active**: Aim for regular exercise, including at least 30 minutes of walking each day to help regulate cholesterol and blood pressure.
- **Quit smoking**: Stopping smoking is one of the most important things you can do to benefit your heart and overall health.

Energy Action Plan – my next steps

It's time to grab your notebook! This is your chance to start taking proactive steps toward better health and wellbeing. What stood out to you in this section? Are you up to date with these key health checks?

Perhaps it's time to book an appointment with your doctor. Or maybe you need to request a copy of your recent results to better understand your health and to stay on top of it. Could this be the moment to make changes to your diet and lifestyle?

Take note of anything that resonated with you and commit to addressing it.

Focus on these three questions to create your SMART objectives:

1. What will I do?
2. How will I do it?
3. When will I do it by?

STEP 3

NUTRITION ESSENTIALS: COMPLETE THE 14-DAY ENERGY BOOST PROGRAMME

The Happy Menopause Energy Clinic in this book is inspired by the experience you'd have working with me in my real-world nutrition clinic, so our next step is to get the basics of your diet right. This will ensure that the energy production chain reaction is activated correctly and runs smoothly. A busy schedule where you're juggling multiple commitments can often mean that good habits go out of the window. There's no doubt that over time this will have a significant impact on your physical and mental energy.

During the perimenopause and menopause, it's more vital than ever that you're eating a carefully balanced diet and looking after yourself. This is a major hormonal transition (just like puberty) and the kinder you are to yourself, the more likely it is that you will have a positive experience.

In this section, we're going to focus on the all-important fuel for energy: macronutrients (proteins, fats and carbohydrates) and water. We'll be dealing with micronutrients in the next chapter. A careful balance of these macronutrients and hydration is absolutely fundamental to our energy levels.

If we don't have enough fuel, or we're not getting the right kind of fuel, this will affect our physical and mental strength, speed and stamina. We'll feel weak and tired. Our brain won't be firing on all cylinders, and we will struggle with memory, focus and concentration. It will be impossible to think creatively or to solve problems and we'll probably be in a pretty bad mood, because positivity, cheerfulness and optimism are very hard to summon up when we feel exhausted.

Here's What We Do First: Fuel Your Energy

In my nutrition clinic, I start by focusing on the correct balance of macronutrients and hydration. It may seem pretty basic, and not as exciting as trying out some miracle superfood to boost our energy, but these simple measures are the absolute foundations of good health. If you start by getting this balance right, your body will be very happy indeed and many niggling issues you've been grappling with could simply melt away.

The macronutrients – proteins, fats and carbohydrates – play a critical role in all our systems. These are the nutrients that we require in large quantities and they influence every physiological and biochemical function in the body. They are also vital for optimal functioning of the mitochondrial pathways that are fundamental to energy production. Simply starting here and getting the balance of the macros right really could make you feel like a whole new woman.

Let's start with a brief explanation of these key dietary pillars that underpin our vitality. This knowledge will help you stay on track when you move on to the really exciting part of this chapter – the 14-day Energy Boost Programme.

My Energy Boost Programme focuses on getting the basics right and could make a world of difference to how you feel in just a few days.

Keep your notebook to hand, jot down anything that resonates with you and remember to create SMART objectives whenever you are prompted to work on your Energy Action Plan (see page 11) to ensure your goals are realistic.

Let's get started with our clinical session by taking a look at each of these macronutrients to see why they're so important.

UNDERSTANDING PROTEIN

I'm starting with protein because it literally is the stuff of life: we are made of protein, and we simply can't function without it. Proteins are complex molecules that consist of building blocks called amino acids.

Protein supports the structure, growth and repair of cells in organs, tissues, bones and connective tissue. It's especially important if we're recovering from illness or injury, and it helps to support strength and stamina. Our skin, hair and nails are all made of a hard form of protein called keratin.

We need proteins to speed up the chemical reactions involved in energy production, digestive function and DNA production. The antibodies powered by our immune function to protect us against infection are actually proteins.

Protein also plays a role in fluid balance and transporting nutrients around the body. Some proteins also function as hormones, such as insulin, which helps to regulate our blood sugar.

How does protein support my energy levels?

Protein is not the body's preferred source fuel for energy, as I explained in Step 1. It will usually only draw on protein for energy if no carbohydrate or fat is available, which may lead to muscle wastage. However, the multi-faceted role of protein means that it gets involved in all sorts of different functions across the body, so it can impact our energy levels in a variety of other ways.

One of these is the role protein plays in maintaining blood sugar balance. The fluctuations of blood sugar can lead to significant energy crashes, which will leave you feeling tired, irritable and unproductive, as well as affecting memory and concentration. This is explored in more detail on pages 114–16.

The amino acids found in protein are used by the body to create key neurotransmitters which regulate mood, memory, focus and concentration. If you're not eating sufficient protein, this will impact your cognitive function. In other words, your brain might not be firing on all cylinders.

Certain amino acids help to increase physical endurance and can enhance sporting performance. They can reduce fatigue, support muscle function and recovery, and improve mental clarity.

Typical signs of a low-protein diet

- Loss of muscle tone
- Hair loss
- Weak or brittle nails
- Brain fog
- Sugar cravings
- Low bone density
- Bad skin
- Slow recovery from injury
- Low mood
- Lack of strength and stamina

Why is protein important during the menopause?

There is no doubt that protein is important for everyone at every stage of life. For women in midlife, it becomes even more of a priority. The drop in oestrogen as we move through the menopause affects us in a number of different ways: we can lose up to 40 per cent of muscle mass and up to 25 per cent of bone density by the time we've gone through the menopause.

Building up our bones and muscles through strength training and resistance work is very important to address this issue. However, we also need protein to feed our bones and muscles.

The hormonal fluctuation around this time can lead to issues such as brain fog, poor memory and problems with concentration. It's also quite common for women to experience thinning hair or weak, splitting nails. If these are concerns for you, you may feel that it's all about the hormones and there's not much you can do. But is that the full picture?

It's important to ensure that you're giving your body the raw materials it needs to do its job. If you're not eating enough protein, then this might be a factor in some of your symptoms.

For example, the role of the amino acids in neurotransmitter function is very important in addressing any issues around mental clarity or low mood. Without these key nutrients, your brain won't be functioning properly, irrespective of your hormonal status.

If your diet is low in protein, your body will prioritize your vital organs, such as your heart, liver or lungs, and send the supplies to them to keep you fit and strong. It won't care that your hair isn't looking great or that your nails keep breaking, because that's not essential to keep you alive!

Why you might be missing out on protein

- You're not eating enough protein with every meal.
- You may not be eating enough complete protein (see page 45).
- Certain digestive disorders can affect protein absorption.
- Kidney or liver dysfunction can also impair protein absorption.

DIETARY SOURCES OF PROTEIN

Protein is made up of a series of amino acids. Nine of these are called essential amino acids, because they can only be acquired through our diet. The body uses these to produce the remaining amino acids that we need for all the different vital functions listed in the previous section.

SOURCES AND FUNCTIONS OF AMINO ACIDS			
Amino acid	**Essential (yes/no)**	**Examples of food sources**	**Functions**
Histidine	Yes	Meat, fish, poultry, soya products, eggs, quinoa, beans	Growth, repair of tissues and production of histamine
Isoleucine	Yes	Eggs, chicken, fish, lentils, cheese, soya protein, almonds, peas	Muscle function, strength and stamina; haemoglobin production; blood sugar regulation
Leucine	Yes	Beef, chicken, salmon, eggs, milk, peanuts, chickpeas/garbanzo beans, lentils	Muscle growth and recovery; regulates blood sugar levels
Lysine	Yes	Red meat, pork, poultry, dairy, soya, quinoa, pumpkin seeds, black beans	Supports collagen formation, calcium absorption and immune function

SOURCES AND FUNCTIONS OF AMINO ACIDS

Amino acid	Essential (yes/no)	Examples of food sources	Functions
Methionine	Yes	Eggs, fish, Brazil nuts, sesame seeds, lean meats	Supports digestion and detoxification
Phenylalanine	Yes	Soya products, beef, chicken, eggs, dairy, tofu, lentils	Precursor to neurotransmitters such as dopamine and adrenaline which regulate mood and mental alertness
Threonine	Yes	Cottage cheese, lentils, fish, poultry, sesame seeds, flaxseed, spirulina	Supports structural proteins such as collagen and elastin; aids in fat metabolism
Tryptophan	Yes	Turkey, chicken, eggs, dairy, oats, chocolate, banana, chia seeds	Precursor to serotonin (the "good mood" neurotransmitter) and melatonin, required for optimal sleep
Valine	Yes	Beef, chicken, peanuts, soya protein, mushrooms, lentils	Aids in muscle growth and recovery; supports energy, endurance and tissue repair

SOURCES AND FUNCTIONS OF AMINO ACIDS

Amino acid	Essential (yes/no)	Examples of food sources	Functions
Alanine	No	Meat, fish, eggs, dairy, wholegrains	Plays a role in energy production and immune system support
Arginine	No	Turkey, pork loin, pumpkin seeds, soya beans, peanuts	Cell growth and development; supports wound healing and immune function
Asparagine	No	Dairy, meat, poultry, eggs, asparagus	Important for protein synthesis, muscle tissue and the nervous system
Aspartic acid	No	Sprouted vegetables, oysters, chicken, eggs, lentils	Plays a role in the citric acid cycle and hormone production
Cysteine	No	Eggs, pork, poultry, broccoli, Brussels sprouts, oats	Precursor to glutathione, a powerful antioxidant which supports detoxification
Glutamic acid	No	Cheese, soy sauce, mushrooms, tomatoes, seaweed	Involved in cognitive function; a precursor to GABA, which is a calming neurotransmitter

SOURCES AND FUNCTIONS OF AMINO ACIDS

Amino acid	Essential (yes/no)	Examples of food sources	Functions
Glutamine	No	Beef, chicken, fish, dairy, spinach, cabbage, lentils	Important for gut health, energy production, memory, focus and concentration
Glycine	No	Gelatine, chicken skin, pork skin, bone broth, tofu, kale	Involved in collagen formation; supports memory and cognitive function
Proline	No	Gelatine, bone broth, dairy, cabbage, soya products	Key component in collagen, aids in skin health and wound healing
Serine	No	Eggs, soya products, fish, lentils, nuts, quinoa	Supports metabolism, immune function and brain signalling
Tyrosine	No	Dairy, turkey, chicken, fish, peanuts, avocado	Supports thyroid hormone function; precursor to dopamine and adrenaline, which regulate mood and mental alertness

Complete proteins

Animal sources of protein (meat, fish, eggs or dairy) are known as complete proteins, because they contain all the essential amino acids that the body needs to synthesize the remaining ones. Most plant proteins, such as pulses, nuts or seeds, contain some but not all the essential amino acids.

This means that if you are following a vegan diet or primarily plant-based diet, you will have to work hard to mix and match the different plant proteins to get what you need in your diet. Soya bean, hemp, buckwheat, chia seed, spirulina and quinoa are examples of complete plant proteins.

How much protein do I need in my diet?

We need to be eating protein with every meal and snack to ensure that we get everything we need. During menopause, we need around 1.0–1.2g of protein per kilo of body weight. For example, a woman weighing 70kg/11 stone would need 70–84g/2½–3oz of protein per day. Aiming for roughly 25g/1oz at breakfast, lunch and dinner should help you keep on track.

This table sets out the protein content of a range of different foods, to give you an idea of the types of foods that you might need to prioritize in your diet to ensure that you're getting all the protein that you require. Don't worry if it looks like a lot of data – if you follow the advice in the 14-Day Energy Boost Programme you'll achieve the right balance. This is just an extra reference tool that you might find useful.

PROTEIN CONTENT OF EVERYDAY FOODS PER 100G

Complete proteins	Incomplete proteins
Meat	**Pulses**
Turkey breast 35g	Chickpeas/garbanzo beans 8.5g
Braised beef 32g	Blackeye beans 8.5g
Steak 30g	Kidney beans 8g
Chicken breast 30g	Lentils 8g
Roasted lamb leg 29g	Peas 6g
Lamb chops 28g	Butter/lima beans 6g
Beef mince 25g	Baked beans 5g
Fish	Broad/fava beans 5g
Salmon 24g	**Nuts**
Canned tuna 24g	Peanuts 25g
Baked cod 23g	Almonds 21g
Grilled haddock 23g	Cashews 20g
Canned sardines 22g	Brazil nuts 14g
Grilled plaice 21g	Walnuts 14g
Mackerel 20g	Hazelnuts 14g
Eggs	**Seeds**
Boiled egg 14g	Pumpkin seeds 24g
Poached egg 13g	Flaxseed 23g

PROTEIN CONTENT OF EVERYDAY FOODS PER 100G

Complete proteins	Incomplete proteins
Dairy	Sunflower seeds 19g
Cheddar cheese 25g	Sesame seeds 18g
Feta cheese 15g	Tahini paste 18g
Cottage cheese 10g	**Other incomplete proteins**
Strained Greek yogurt 9g	Wholemeal bread 9g
Full-fat plain yogurt 6g	White bread 8g
Low-fat plain yogurt 5g	Wholegrain pasta 5g
Greek-style yogurt 6g	Oats 4.5g
Milk (whole, semi- or skimmed) 3.5g	White pasta 4g
Soya	Brown rice 3.6g
Boiled edamame soya bean 14g	White rice 2.8g
Firm tofu 8g	Avocado 2g
Silken tofu 4g	Mushrooms 1.4g
Other complete proteins	
Spirulina 57g	
Hemp 31g	
Chia seeds 16g	
Quinoa 4.4g	

CASE STUDY: The power of protein – Catherine's story

Catherine, 56, consulted me for advice to improve her energy, sleep and overall wellbeing. An analysis of her diet revealed that she wasn't eating enough protein and that her diet lacked complete protein. I also felt she would benefit from more animal protein, as some people absorb this more effectively than plant protein.

I asked her to increase protein at breakfast, add animal protein to her lunch and ensure a good portion of protein with her dinner.

After just eight days, she reported feeling much stronger and more resilient. Her energy was more consistent, and best of all, the quality of her sleep had improved. She found it much easier to get back to sleep if she woke up during the night, and her sleep was more restful and peaceful overall. This is such a great example of the power of protein.

Easy ways to increase protein in your diet

- Eat a portion of protein-rich food with every meal and snack.
- Whenever you're about to eat something, ask yourself where the protein is. If it's not there, add it!
- Make sure you're eating at least one complete protein every day, to access the essential amino acids you need.
- Add 2 tablespoons of seeds or chopped nuts to your morning cereal. Milk or yogurt alone isn't always enough, but together they make a protein-packed start to your day.
- Stir a heaped tablespoon of ground flaxseed into vegetable soup to boost the protein content.

- Opt for authentic strained Greek yogurt, which is richer in protein than Greek-style yogurt.
- Include protein in any snacks: houmous, unsweetened nut butter and raw, unsalted nuts or seeds.
- If you follow a plant-based diet, be sure to rotate your protein sources to access all the amino acids you need.

Energy Action Plan – my next steps

Take a moment to reflect on what you've learned about protein. Has this section given you food for thought? What stood out to you the most? Think about some simple steps you can take to ensure you're eating enough protein and jot them down in your notebook – you'll be putting them into practice very soon!

Focus on these three questions to create your SMART objectives:

1. What will I do?
2. How will I do it?
3. When will I do it by?

UNDERSTANDING FAT

Many midlife women can be nervous about fat. We're the generation who grew up with the low-fat message being drummed into us as the fundamental route to weight loss. In my nutrition clinic, I regularly encounter a reluctance from women to eat foods that they perceive as being high in fat, because they're worried that this will affect their weight.

Despite the bad press, good-quality fat is actually our friend on so many levels. It has multiple vital functions in the body, is critical to our health, and we avoid it at our peril.

Fats fall into three categories: saturated, polyunsaturated and mono-unsaturated. Each type is very important for our health, which is why we need a combination of all three in our diet.

The body uses saturated fat to make cholesterol, which is a key constituent of every cell in the body, in the correct amount. We need cholesterol to make sex hormones, to synthesize vitamin D from sunlight, and to produce cortisol, which manages our stress response but also has a role in the sleep–wake cycle, metabolism, blood sugar balance and blood pressure regulation.

Poly- and monounsaturated fats, chiefly made up of the essential fatty acids omega-3, -6 and -9, support cardiovascular function, promote hormone balance and skin health, and are crucial for the optimal functioning of the brain and nervous system.

We also need fat to store the fat-soluble vitamins A, D, E and K, so that we can use them as required.

How does fat support my energy levels?

Fat is a very dense source of energy for the body and contains twice as much energy per gram as carbohydrate or protein. If no carbohydrate is available, or if we are involved in a prolonged medium-intensity activity, the body will draw on fat for energy through a process called lipolysis. This breaks down the fat into fatty acids and glycerol, which are transported to the mitochondria in our cells and used for ATP production. It's particularly helpful as a source of fuel for endurance exercise.

The brain requires essential fatty acids, such as omega-3, to support the structural integrity and fluidity of cell membranes. This ensures the optimal function of neurons and neurotransmitters, which underpin mental clarity, concentration, memory and mood.

Essential fatty acids also have an anti-inflammatory role, helping to protect the brain against oxidation and inflammation, which can impair cognitive function.

Typical signs of a low-fat diet

- Dry or flaky skin
- Brittle or dull hair
- Stiff or sore joints
- Menstrual problems
- Poor concentration and memory
- Low mood
- Vitamin D deficiency
- Lack of energy
- Small bumps on the skin on the back of the arms

Why is fat important during the menopause?

The fluctuation and subsequent decline in sex hormones during the perimenopause and menopause make fat a very important nutrient for the midlife woman. The body needs dietary fat to produce sex hormones, which is why this is no time for a very low-fat diet. We need to give our body the raw materials to produce and maintain the balance of hormones we need, otherwise, we run the risk of experiencing more severe symptoms.

The role of the essential fatty acids in supporting emotional wellbeing and cognitive function is also key during this stage of life. Many women experience issues with mood swings, anxiety or brain fog, so it's very important to ensure that your diet includes plenty of poly- and monounsaturated fats.

Heart health is also a consideration. There is a very strong evidence base for the importance of omega fatty acids in maintaining our cardiovascular health, supporting cardiac function, promoting healthy blood vessels and regulating cholesterol levels.

Fat also nourishes our skin, helping it to retain moisture and flexibility. It's common to experience dry skin and a loss of elasticity during menopause.

The anti-inflammatory properties of essential fatty acids help to keep your joints from aching and feeling stiff, which can become more common with the drop in oestrogen.

Why you might be missing out on fat

- You're avoiding fat in your diet and consciously opting for low-fat products in the supermarket.
- Low levels of bile acids or a lack of pancreatic enzymes can impair fat absorption.
- Excessive levels of saturated fats or artificial trans fats can block the action of essential fatty acids.
- Too much omega-6 in your diet can affect the action of omega-3.

DIETARY SOURCES OF FAT

Fats are called saturated or unsaturated based on their chemical structure and the amount of double bonds between the carbon atoms in the fatty acid chains. All foods that contain fat will include a combination of saturated, polyunsaturated and monounsaturated fats, although the ratio will be different. For example, red meat will be higher in saturated and lower in unsaturated fat, whereas the opposite applies to oily fish.

Saturated fats

Saturated fats are mostly found in animal foods, especially meat and dairy, although coconut or palm oil are examples of plant sources. These fats are generally solid at room temperature and are more stable when cooked at high temperatures compared to unsaturated fats.

Unsaturated fats

Monounsaturated and polyunsaturated fats are found in abundance in fish, nuts and seeds, and are usually liquid at room temperature. However, the oils from unsaturated fats can be more volatile when cooked and may require gentler heat due to their lower smoking points. When heated to very high temperatures, they can lose some of their beneficial properties.

Omega-9 is perhaps the most well-known monounsaturated fat. Olive oil is an excellent source, with about 83 per cent of it being omega-9. Avocado is another great source.

Polyunsaturated fats primarily consist of omega-3 and omega-6, both of which are essential fatty acids. These are called "essential" because the body cannot produce them and must obtain them through diet. Omega-3 and omega-6 fats are found in abundance in oily fish, flaxseed, and various other seeds and nuts.

Trans fats

These are a type of unsaturated fat with a chemical structure that makes them behave more like saturated fats. While very small amounts of trans fats occur naturally, the primary concern is artificial trans fats. These are created through a process of hydrogenation, which alters the chemical structure of the fat and extends the shelf life of processed products.

Artificial trans fats have been heavily restricted or banned in many countries, including the USA and the UK, due to their established link to heart disease, type 2 diabetes and other chronic health conditions. It's still important to watch out for them, especially in ultra-processed foods, some baked goods and certain fast foods.

When checking food labels, look for "partially hydrogenated oils" in the ingredients list, as these are a key source of trans fats. Be cautious of foods that list these oils, as they can contribute to your intake of unhealthy fats.

How much fat do I need in my diet?

We need to be eating around 70g/2½oz of fat each day, which breaks down like this:

Saturated fats

The daily recommended amount for women consuming a standard diet of 2,000 calories per day is a maximum of 20g/¾oz. This is best consumed via good-quality sources of fat, such as meat from grass-fed cattle, organic or artisan dairy produce, or coconut oil, for example. Deep-fried foods are best avoided due to the risk of trans fats.

Unsaturated fats

At least 50g/1¾oz per day should come from poly- and monounsaturated fats. The ratio of omega-6 to omega-3 should be between 4:1 and 2:1, to achieve the correct balance. However, in the Western diet, the ratio is more likely to be between 8:1 and 25:1, due to an overreliance on processed foods, such as potato chips, which are often made with vegetable oils that are high in omega-6.

The tables below provide a selection of everyday foods that are good sources of different types of fats.

You might find it useful to see the balance of saturated and unsaturated fats in some common foods, especially if you feel the need to focus a bit more carefully on one or the other. That said, you don't need to spend too much time here – unless you enjoy delving into the stats! In the 14-Day Energy Boost Programme, I'll be guiding you toward achieving the correct balance.

This table focuses on animal fats. I've divided it into three columns so you can easily see how the fats break down into saturated, monounsaturated and polyunsaturated types. For example, you can see that red meat and cheese are higher in saturated fats than oily fish, which is an excellent source of unsaturated fat.

FAT CONTENT OF EVERYDAY ANIMAL PRODUCTS PER 100G		
Food type	**Saturated fat**	**Monounsaturated fat**	**Polyunsaturated fat**
Meat			
Bacon	8g	10g	3g
Beef mince	6g	6g	0.6g
Braising steak	4g	4g	0.6g
Pork	4g	4g	1.4g
Ham	4g	5g	2g
Lamb	4g	4g	0.6g
Lean rump steak	2g	2g	0.5g
Chicken	2g	3.5g	1.5g
Turkey	0.7g	0.7g	0.5g
Fish			
Mackerel	5g	8g	5g
Salmon	3g	6g	5g
Smoked salmon	2g	3g	3g
Sardines	2.5g	2.5g	3g
Tuna	0.3g	0.2g	0.5g
White fish	0.1g	0.1g	0.1g

Food type	Saturated fat	Monounsaturated fat	Polyunsaturated fat
FAT CONTENT OF EVERYDAY ANIMAL PRODUCTS PER 100G			
Dairy			
Butter	52g	21g	3g
Spreadable butter	34g	30g	10g
Double cream	33g	14g	2g
Single cream	12g	5g	0.6g
Cheddar	21g	9g	1g
Parmesan	19g	7g	1g
Halloumi	17g	6g	1g
Mozzarella	14g	5g	0.8g
Feta	13g	4g	0.6g
Full-fat milk	2g	1g	0.1g
Semi-skimmed milk	1g	0.4g	Traces
Skimmed milk	0.1g	0.1g	Traces
Full-fat natural yogurt	2g	0.7g	0.1g
Low-fat natural yogurt	0.7g	0.2g	Traces
Eggs	3g	4g	1.5g

The next table provides the same breakdown for plant-based sources of fat. I've rearranged the columns here, starting with polyunsaturates, as these foods tend to be much higher in unsaturated fats.

Food type	Polyunsaturated fat	Monounsaturated fat	Saturated fat
FAT CONTENT OF EVERYDAY PLANT PRODUCTS PER 100G			
Nuts			
Walnuts	47g	11g	7g
Brazil nuts	25g	22g	17g
Peanuts	13g	22g	9g
Almonds	11g	38g	4g
Cashews	9g	29g	10g
Hazelnuts	7g	49g	5g
Seeds			
Flaxseed	29g	6g	4g
Sunflower seeds	28g	11g	7g
Sesame seeds	26g	22.1g	10.5g
Chia seeds	25g	2g	3g
Pumpkin seeds	18g	11g	7g
Oils			
Walnut oil	70g	16g	8g
Sunflower oil	63g	20g	12g
Rapeseed/canola oil	29g	59g	6g
Palm oil	10g	37g	48g
Olive oil	8g	73g	14g
Coconut oil	1.5g	6g	86g
Other			
Tofu	2g	8g	4g
Avocado	2g	12g	4g

Finding the right omega-3 and omega-6 balance

A diet rich in omega fatty acids is crucial for overall health. However, achieving the right balance between omega-3 and omega-6 is equally important for optimal health and reducing inflammation. The ideal ratio is thought to be around 4:1 (omega-6 to omega-3), but modern diets often contain far more omega-6, which can tip the scales and contribute to inflammation.

This table helps you assess the approximate ratio of omega-3 to omega-6 in foods high in polyunsaturated fats. You'll notice that many of these foods contain significantly more omega-6, which can cause an imbalance in the typical diet. To counteract this, aim to include foods rich in omega-3 several times a week, such as oily fish, flaxseed and chia seeds. This can help maintain the recommended omega-3 levels and support overall wellbeing.

OMEGA-3 AND OMEGA-6 CONTENT OF FOODS HIGH IN POLYUNSATURATES

Food type	Omega-3 content per 100g	Omega-6 content per 100g
Oily fish		
Mackerel	2.7g	0.3g
Salmon	2.6g	0.4g
Sardines	1.5g	0.1g
Nuts		
Walnuts	9g	38g
Brazil nuts	0.1g	20.6g
Almonds	0.1g	11g
Seeds		
Flaxseed	22g	5.9g
Chia seeds	18g	6.7g
Sesame seeds	0.2g	21.4g
Sunflower seeds	0.1g	23.1g
Pumpkin seeds	0.1g	19g
Oils		
Walnut oil	10g	52g
Sunflower oil	0.1g	63g
Rapeseed oil	9g	20g

CASE STUDY: Why fat is your friend – Amanda's story

Amanda, 47, came to my clinic seeking advice on weight loss. She was also struggling with low energy, joint pain, dry skin and dull hair. She was constantly hungry and snacking, which was inevitably impacting her weight. It was immediately clear that we needed to address the amount of fat in her diet, as these are classic signs of a low-fat or no-fat eating pattern.

At first, she was sceptical about including more fat in her diet, but I explained that it could actually help with both weight loss and energy. Healthy fats are filling, keep you satisfied for longer and provide a valuable energy source.

She agreed to swap her usual low-fat options, such as yogurt and cottage cheese, for full-fat versions. She also started eating oily fish three times a week and added omega-3-rich raw nuts and seeds to her daily meals, and we discussed some targeted supplements.

By the end of our 12-week programme, Amanda had stopped snacking altogether and was well on her way to achieving her weight-loss goal. She had more energy and her skin was glowing, proving that the right fats can make a difference.

Easy Ways to Increase Healthy Fats in Your Diet

- Eat oily fish, such as salmon, mackerel or sardines, three times a week.
- Add 2 tablespoons of flaxseed or chia seeds to your morning cereal.
- Drizzle a tablespoon of olive oil over your vegetables when you serve them (unless you've already cooked them in olive oil).

- Enjoy unsweetened nut butter on wholemeal toast, instead of jam or honey.
- Stir a spoonful of unsweetened nut butter into porridge, oatmeal or a smoothie – that's a double-whammy of creaminess and good fats.
- Choose full-fat organic dairy products over low-fat options.
- Use the whole egg, rather than just the egg white, in an omelette, because the yolk is where all the lovely fat resides.
- Add coconut milk to soups, smoothies or curries.
- Eat meat from pasture-fed cattle: studies have shown that it contains higher levels of omega-3 fatty acids.

Energy Action Plan – my next steps

Were you surprised by anything in this section? Perhaps you feel more positive toward fats than you did before. Take a moment to think about whether you're consuming enough of the right types of fats and consider the steps you could take to improve this. Jot down any ideas in your notebook – they'll soon be helpful as you dive into the Energy Boost Programme.

Focus on these three questions to create your SMART objectives:

1. What will I do?
2. How will I do it?
3. When will I do it by?

UNDERSTANDING CARBOHYDRATE

Carbohydrate is the body's primary source of energy, which is why a very-low-carb diet won't be helpful if you experience physical or mental fatigue.

Carbohydrate is found exclusively in plant foods, apart from milk and milk products, which contain a sugar called lactose. We often think of carbs as starchy foods, such as bread, rice or pasta, but it's important to remember that fruit, vegetables and pulses are carbohydrates too.

Carbohydrates naturally fall into two groups: simple and complex carbohydrate. However, with the advent of food processing and manufacturing, there is a third category, known as refined carbohydrate.

TYPES OF CARBOHYDRATE

Category	Description	Examples
Simple carbohydrate	Rapidly digestible carbohydrate, made of one or two sugars (monosaccharides or disaccharides). Its simple structure allows it to be rapidly processed and absorbed into the bloodstream, which can lead to blood sugar spikes and energy crashes.	Glucose, fructose (fruit sugar), lactose (milk sugar), sucrose (table sugar), honey, jam, maple syrup, high-fructose corn syrup

TYPES OF CARBOHYDRATE		
Category	**Description**	**Examples**
Complex carbohydrate	Longer chains of sugar called polysaccharides. They also include starch and fibre. This more complex structure means that they take longer to digest and the release of sugar into the bloodstream is more gradual. This helps to maintain the correct blood sugar balance and allows for more sustained energy.	Wholegrains, e.g. brown rice, wholemeal bread, wholewheat pasta, quinoa, oats, bran; pulses, e.g. lentils, chickpeas/garbanzo beans, beans; starchy vegetables, e.g. corn, sweet potato, squash; whole fruits with an edible skin; nuts and seeds
Refined carbohydrate	Processed carbohydrate that has been mostly stripped of the fibre and other nutrients during the manufacturing process. This leaves the sugar and digestible starch, which is processed more rapidly.	White bread, white rice, white pasta; white flour; pastries, cakes and other baked goods; sugary breakfast cereals; sodas and sugary drinks; chocolate and other confectionery

The fibre found in complex carbohydrate plays a very important role in our health and wellbeing, even though only a small proportion can be broken down and digested, because dietary fibre is mostly resistant to the body's digestive enzymes. Much of the fibre we eat passes through the digestive tract and ends up in our stools, but along the way it does some very important work.

Fibre helps to feed the beneficial bacteria in the gut which are so important for our digestive health and immune function; it supports the healthy formation and passage of stools, reducing the risk of constipation and haemorrhoids; it also promotes hormone balance (see below).

How does carbohydrate support my energy levels?

Carbohydrate is a quick-and-easy source of energy for the body. It's the main source of blood glucose, which is the principal source of fuel for every cell in the body, and is the only source of energy for the brain. Low levels of carbohydrate will leave us feeling tired and lethargic, significantly affecting physical performance as well as impairing our thought processes, focus, concentration and memory.

Both simple and complex carbohydrate (excluding fibre) are converted into glucose. This is then used immediately to provide energy or stored in the liver as glycogen for use in the future.

If we eat more carbohydrate than we need for energy or that the liver can store, any excess will be stored as fat cells. This is why high levels of carbohydrate can be a common culprit in weight gain.

Although fibre isn't used as a source of fuel, it nevertheless indirectly supports our energy levels, because of the key role it plays in helping optimal digestion and nutrient absorption. As we have seen in Chapter 1, many key macro- and micronutrients are very important for energy and if we don't absorb these nutrients effectively, the chain reaction of energy production will be impacted.

Typical signs of a low-carb diet

- Fatigue
- Headaches
- Dizziness or weakness
- Lack of stamina
- Constipation
- Digestive problems
- Sugar cravings
- Brain fog
- Irritability
- Short-term memory issues
- Energy crashes

Why is carbohydrate important during the menopause?

Low energy and fatigue are common issues during the menopause, so it's important to ensure that you're accessing the quick-and-easy source of fuel that carbohydrate provides.

While the body can draw on fat as an alternative to carbohydrate if sources are low, this is not the case for the brain, which is entirely reliant on glucose for the energy it needs to help us keep firing on all cylinders. If you're experiencing issues with brain fog, low mood or anxiety, it's important to ensure that you're feeding your brain with the fuel it needs.

Excessive levels of simple or refined carbohydrate may contribute to weight gain, but complex carbohydrate can help you in lots of different ways.

It will support sustained energy, keeping you going during a busy day and reducing those sugar cravings that can lead to snacking between meals.

The fibre found in complex carbs will support optimal digestive function, reducing issues such as bloating, constipation or loose stools. It also helps to regulate cholesterol levels, which become more of a concern as we transition through menopause.

Fibre will support the correct hormone balance, by binding itself to excess oestrogen in the gut and excreting it via the stools. This is especially important during the perimenopause when fluctuating hormone levels can be an issue: excessive levels of oestrogen during this phase may lead to heavier, longer or more painful periods.

Carbohydrate could even help with the quality of our hair. The hair follicles are among the fastest reproducing cells in the body, which means that they use up a lot of energy. If you're following a low-carb diet, this may lead to thinning hair, which is a common problem for some women in mid- and later life.

Why you might be missing out on carbohydrate

- You're following a low-carb or no-carb weight-loss regime.
- You're not eating enough vegetables.
- Your diet is high in processed foods or ready meals.
- You opt for refined carbohydrates, such as white bread, white rice or white pasta.
- Certain digestive disorders can affect the body's ability to break down and absorb carbohydrate.

DIETARY SOURCES OF CARBOHYDRATE

Carbohydrates encompass a broad range of food from a sweet potato or a tomato to a chocolate bar or a slice of bread. To maximize the energy-supporting action of carbohydrate and to ensure a sustained effect over a period of hours, it's preferable to focus on complex carbohydrates that are rich in fibre. If this is a big change for you, it's wise to build up the fibre content slowly so your digestion can adjust to this. Fibre can be very stimulating for the gut, which may cause some initial bloating if you're over-enthusiastic with your approach!

Of course you can still enjoy the occasional indulgence – there's nothing wrong with having a sugary treat from time to time. But if sugar is a regular fixture of your diet, this will be affecting your blood sugar balance and is likely to be the culprit behind the energy slumps you experience. See page 113 for more information on the link between blood sugar balance and energy.

Cold carbs keep you fuller!

Cooking and cooling rice, pasta or potatoes creates resistant starch, which helps sustain blood sugar levels for longer. This is why a pasta, potato or rice salad can keep you feeling fuller – even when made with white rice or pasta!

How much carbohydrate do I need in my diet?
Fibre

Adults should be aiming for 30g/1oz of fibre every day, although many people consume nearer 20g/¾oz, which simply isn't enough to support a healthy digestion. The easiest way to get the fibre we need is to opt for wholegrain foods and to aim to eat five different vegetables every day.

At breakfast time, opt for 1–2 slices of wholemeal bread (plus a protein source) or around 40g of wholegrain cereal, with nuts or seeds for an extra fibre boost. Think of your lunch and dinner as quadrants: one quarter is a protein-rich food, such as meat, fish, tofu or pulses. Foods that contain protein also contain fat, which covers off that requirement. The remaining three quarters will be made up of different forms of carbohydrate. This approach helps maintain the ideal balance of macronutrients. Each quarter of the meal you serve should be approximately the size of a fist, ensuring an appropriate portion and a balanced mix of macronutrients to support your energy.

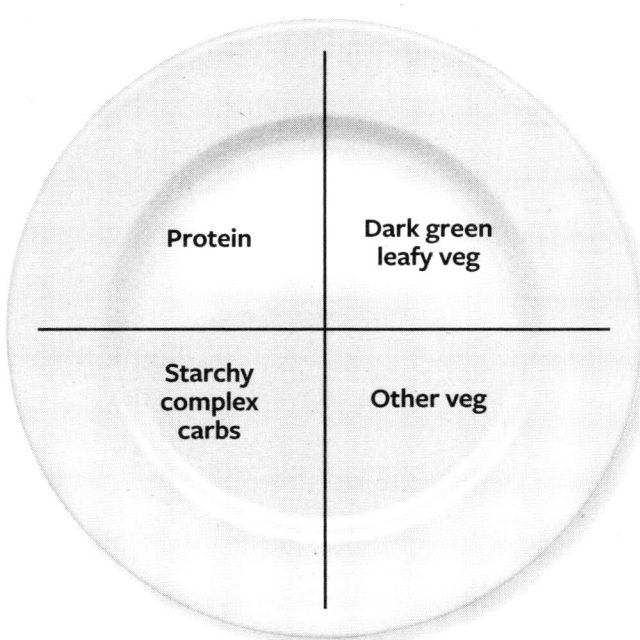

Meal structure at lunch and dinner

Free sugar

It's recommended that we shouldn't eat more than 30g/1oz of free sugar every day. Free sugars are sugars that have been added to a food; they also include honey, syrup and fruit juices or smoothies. Sugars found in whole fruits, vegetables and milk are not considered free sugars. See page 119 for advice on understanding sugar labelling.

You can see in the table below the average amount of fibre in a range of everyday foods. This should help you plan your meals in a way that optimizes your intake of fibre. I'll be helping with this when you start the Energy Boost Programme.

FIBRE CONTENT OF EVERYDAY STARCHY FOODS PER PORTION

Food type	Fibre	Carbohydrate
White bread (per slice)	1g	19g
Wholemeal bread (per slice)	2.5g	16g
White rice (per 100g)	0.4g	30g
Brown rice (per 100g)	1.8g	23g
White pasta (per 100g)	1.1g	31g
Wholewheat pasta (per 100g)	3.7g	28g
Overnight oats (per 40g)	4.2g	10.8g
Cooked oats (per 40g)	0.9g	4.8g
Shredded wheat-type cereal (per 40g)	4.2g	28g

FIBRE CONTENT OF EVERYDAY STARCHY FOODS PER PORTION

Food type	Fibre	Carbohydrate
Wheat biscuit-type cereal (per 40g)	3g	29g
Bran flakes (per 40g)	5g	29g
Baked potato with skin (per 100g)	1.4g	23g
Baked sweet potato with skin (per 100g)	3g	20g
Roast potato (per 100g)	1.1g	26g
Quinoa (per 100g)	2.8g	21g

FIBRE CONTENT OF EVERYDAY VEGETABLES PER 100G

Vegetable	Fibre	Carbohydrate
Peas	4.5g	10g
Cabbage	2.6g	3g
Spinach	2.4g	3g
Broccoli	2.3g	3g
Carrot	2g	7g
Mixed salad leaves	1.3g	1.4g
Tomato	1g	3g

FIBRE CONTENT OF EVERYDAY FRUIT PER 100G

Fruit	Fibre	Carbohydrate
Raspberries	2.5g	5g
Pear	1.6g	11g
Blueberries	1.5g	9g
Apple	1.3g	11g
Satsuma/clementine	1.2g	9.6g
Banana	0.8g	20g

Easy ways to increase complex carbohydrate in your diet

- Swap white starch, e.g. white bread, white rice or white pasta, for brown starch, e.g. wholemeal bread, brown rice or wholewheat pasta.
- Aim to eat a least five different vegetables every day.
- Add chopped fresh fruit and seeds to your morning cereal.
- Add pulses to dishes such as casseroles, soups or curries.
- Eat potatoes with the skin on.
- Keep a stock of frozen veg in the freezer to draw on as required.
- Add beans or chickpeas/garbanzo beans to salads.
- Snack on nuts and seeds.
- Choose fruits with an edible skin.

Juice: a hidden sugar trap!

A 250ml/9fl oz/1 cup glass of carton orange juice contains as much as 6 teaspoons of sugar! Opt for whole fruit instead to get the nutrients without the sugar spike.

CASE STUDY: The fibre fix – Sarah's story

Sarah, 51, came to my clinic struggling with bloating and constipation, which were making her feel sluggish and miserable. Her diet was high in refined sugars and starch: she ate a lot of white bread, rice and pasta, and had a weakness for chocolate and other sugary treats.

The first thing we needed to focus on was fibre, as it's crucial for regular and healthy digestive function. I recommended that Sarah aim for four different portions of vegetables every day – two with lunch and two with dinner, or one as a snack (e.g. carrot sticks with houmous). In addition, I advised swapping to brown bread, rice and pasta to boost fibre intake, and also increasing her hydration.

Constipation can be a complex issue, and this was just the first step. We worked together over several weeks to fully address her concerns. However, after just two weeks of making these changes, Sarah already experienced a significant reduction in bloating, and her bowel movements were becoming more regular.

Energy Action Plan – my next steps

What insights did you gain from this section? Are you getting enough fibre in your diet? Maybe you feel that you're consuming too much sugar or refined carbohydrate. Take a moment to note any simple adjustments you could make to promote a healthier balance in your diet. This will be very helpful as you embark on the 14-day Energy Boost Programme.

Focus on these three questions to create your SMART objectives:

1. What will I do?
2. How will I do it?
3. When will I do it by?

UNDERSTANDING HYDRATION

Water is the essence of life and vital to our survival. Over 50 per cent of the female body is made up of water and we need to drink it every day, because the body can't store it. Every single bodily system, as well as all our cells, tissues, muscles, organs and bones, requires water to function correctly. Even mild dehydration can rapidly affect our health, wellbeing and performance in many ways. In fact, studies have shown that just 2 per cent dehydration significantly affects physical performance and cognitive function.

How does water support my energy levels?

Water plays a crucial role in generating energy because we need it to transport oxygen around the body to support the production of the ATP energy storage units in each body cell.

What's more, 75 per cent of the brain is made up of water and if we're not drinking enough, this will affect our memory, concentration and creativity. It can also lead to confusion and irritability.

Dehydration reduces blood volume, which means the heart has to work harder to circulate oxygen and nutrients around the body. This will affect strength and stamina.

Our physical performance and endurance will be reduced by dehydration, and if our muscles are starved of water, this will cause cramping and affect muscle recovery after training.

Typical signs of dehydration

- Headaches
- Fatigue
- Lethargy
- Confusion
- Constipation
- Dry or rough skin
- Dry eyes

- Dizziness
- Muscle cramps
- Thirst
- Dark urine
- Dry mouth
- Low blood pressure

Why is water important during the menopause?

The multifaceted role of water in the body means that dehydration is likely to exacerbate most of the symptoms of the menopause.

Dehydration will affect cognitive function, contributing to issues of brain fog and poor memory, which can already be troubling for some women during the perimenopause. It's also a major factor in fatigue and loss of strength and stamina.

Dry skin and vaginal dryness are common early warning signs of menopause, and again these will be aggravated if you're not drinking enough water.

Water is essential for bone renewal and remodelling. The drop in oestrogen around the menopause affects this process, which can increase the risk of low bone density. It's important to ensure that a lack of hydration isn't getting in the way of building strong bones.

Dehydration could also contribute to the common symptom of stiff and sore joints, because of the role it plays in the production of synovial fluid that keeps our joints lubricated.

Urinary tract infections (UTIs) can become more common at this stage of life. The change in oestrogen levels affects the pH (acid–alkaline) balance of the vagina. It is naturally an acidic environment, which protects us against infection, but the loss of acidity during menopause can make us more vulnerable to UTIs. Even without the hormonal changes of the menopause, dehydration is a common cause of these infections. From perimenopause on, it's even more important to keep well hydrated.

Menstrual migraine becomes more common for some women during the perimenopause and these headaches will be worsened by dehydration.

How much water should I drink?

This is a question I'm asked all the time! The answer isn't clear cut. It really depends on your age, build, state of health, level of physical activity and the temperature of your environment. This is why it will be different for each person.

I always find the mention of 6–8 glasses of water each day pretty meaningless. How big is the glass? Who knows?!

The general recommendation for women is about 2.7 litres/0.7 gallons/11.5 cups per day, which can be consumed as water, other drinks or food. About 20 per cent will come from food, so you're probably looking at about 2 litres/0.5 gallons/8.5 cups per day from drinks.

However this is still very approximate because of the factors listed above and it will be personal to you.

Thirst isn't always a helpful indicator of dehydration. Some people don't have a very active thirst mechanism or are not always aware of their thirst, so may become dehydrated without realizing it.

The best and most individual approach to assessing your hydration is to keep an eye on the colour of your urine. It should be a pale straw colour. If it is darker than this, you are likely to be dehydrated.

DIETARY SOURCES OF WATER

The lists of foods in the tables below could help you optimize your hydration, especially if you find it hard to drink enough water.

WATER CONTENT OF EVERYDAY FRUITS PER 100G	
Watermelon	92ml
Strawberries	91ml
Oranges	88ml
Apples	86ml
Blueberries	84ml
Grapes	81ml

WATER CONTENT OF EVERYDAY VEGETABLES PER 100G

Cucumber	96ml
Lettuce (especially romaine and iceberg varieties)	95ml
Celery	95ml
Courgette/zucchini	94ml
Spinach	93ml
Broccoli	89ml
Carrots	88ml

WATER CONTENT OF PROTEIN SOURCES PER 100G

Whole milk	87ml
Plain yogurt	85ml
Egg	75ml
Chicken breast	65ml
Salmon	68ml
White fish	65ml
Tinned tuna or sardines	65ml
Beef	55ml
Tofu	76ml
Lentils (cooked)	70ml
Chickpeas (cooked)	60ml
Kidney beans (cooked)	73ml

CASE STUDY: Hydration to the rescue – Hannah's story

Hannah, 42, had been suffering from lifelong headaches and migraines when she came to my clinic. Over the years, she had learned to manage them using various strategies. However, as she entered perimenopause, the frequency and severity of her headaches increased, likely due to the hormonal fluctuations during this stage of life.

To help regulate the situation, we implemented a hormone-balancing diet. I also advised her to adjust her hydration habits, as dehydration can be a major trigger for both headaches and migraines. Hannah had been sipping water throughout the day, but some studies suggest that drinking regular large doses of water, rather than sipping constantly, can be more effective.

I recommended she drink eight glasses containing 220ml/7¾fl oz/1 cup of mineral water throughout the day as her baseline for hydration. By the next session, the severity and frequency of her headaches had already decreased by over 50 per cent. The power of water is immense!

Easy ways to improve your hydration

- Set a hydration routine: drink a glass of water as soon as you wake up, then use a water bottle with time markers to remind you to sip throughout the day.
- If you find water is boring, try adding slices of fruit, cucumber, basil or mint to your jug or bottle, to add flavour. Sparkling water with a dash of lime or elderflower cordial adds a celebratory touch to your drink.
- Eat more of the hydrating fruit and vegetables from the tables above.
- Choose soups or broths, as these have a high water content.

- Link water to other daily habits, e.g. drink a glass before a meal or get a drink when you take a break.
- Herbal teas are a great way to drink more water. And even though coffee and tea are mild diuretics, you will retain more fluid than you lose when you drink them.
- Distribute bottles of water around your environment, so there is always an option to hydrate, e.g. leave a bottle in your car, in your bag, by your desk and by the bed.
- If you tend to forget to drink, consider a hydration app or setting timers on your phone to help remind you.

Energy Action Plan – my next steps

Are you consistently staying hydrated or is there room for improvement? Reviewing your fluid intake could be an eye-opener, and ensuring adequate hydration may significantly impact your energy levels.

Create a hydration section in your notebook and list any simple steps you can take to boost your water consumption.

Focus on these three questions to create your SMART objectives:

1. What will I do?
2. How will I do it?
3. When will I do it by?

YOUR 14-DAY ENERGY BOOST PROGRAMME

The previous section explained in detail the importance of the different macronutrients and optimal hydration. Now it's time to put all that useful information into practice by doing the 14-day Energy Boost Programme, before you move onto the energy quizzes in the next chapter.

You may be tempted to skip ahead, but it's important to complete the programme first because much of the physical and mental fatigue you experience may be reduced, or even resolved, by taking in the correct balance of macronutrients and water.

Any lingering issues can then be addressed in the next chapter by working your way through the energy quizzes which focus on potential micronutrient and functional imbalances.

Taking a step-by-step approach is much more likely to help you identify the specific causes of your energy deficit. It will also make the process much more manageable – ideal for the busy and tired midlife woman!

Before you start

Record a score out of 10 in your notebook for each of these areas that can be affected by fatigue: physical energy, strength, stamina, memory, concentration, mental clarity. It's important to write down the scores, because it's very easy to forget how you felt before, once your energy starts to improve. This record will give you something to compare against when you score yourself at the end of the programme.

Score		
0 1 2 3 4 5 6 7 8 9 10		
Very bad		Very good

EATING FOR ENERGY

This programme builds on all the principles outlined above and is designed to help you get the right balance of macronutrients in your diet. Over the next 14 days, you'll follow the guidance provided here. In return, you should start to notice improvements in your energy levels fairly quickly.

You don't need to follow the plan rigidly or eat every meal exactly as described, unless you want to. These are suggestions for you to adapt according to your preferences. You can use the food tables above to stay aligned with your macro goals and draw on your insights from each section to guide your choices.

However, there are a few key guidelines that are non-negotiable. Whatever meals you choose to plan over the next 14 days, make sure that you stick to these essential points.

Energy boost guidelines

1. Three proper meals a day and no snacking.
2. Protein and fibre with every meal.
3. Avoid refined carbohydrates and sugary foods.
4. At least four portions of vegetables every day.
5. Limit fruit to a maximum of two portions per day.
6. Remember to follow the portion sizes shown in the quadrant diagram (see page 69).
7. Hydrate yourself throughout the day.
8. No more than two caffeinated drinks, such as tea or coffee, per day.
9. Eliminate alcohol completely for 14 days.

Energy boost tips for success

1. **Acclimatize your body**

   If this programme isn't so very different from the way you eat most of the time, it's fine to plunge in straightaway. However, if caffeine, alcohol, sugar or processed foods feature regularly in your diet, it would be wise to ease yourself in gently. A sudden change to your diet can be a bit of a shock to the system. These types of foods can be very addictive and it's not unusual to experience unpleasant withdrawal symptoms, such as headaches, fatigue or aching joints if you eliminate them all in one go. A sensible approach would be to reduce your consumption of these foods gradually over about a week, so that your body has had time to adjust before you get going with the programme. You'll benefit much more from the changes if you take it a step at a time.

2. **It's all in the planning**

o Have a good read through the whole chapter before you start, so you can really get to grips with the key principles of the programme.

o Choose a sensible time to start: it can be helpful to pick a 14-day period where you don't have a lot of social engagements, heavy commitments at work or travel planned. You don't have to do this, but it can make adjusting to your new regime a bit easier.

o Get your notebook out and plan the meals for your first week. Doing this will make life so much easier. You can use the meal suggestion table below for some foodie inspiration, or stick with your trusted favourites, making tweaks to ensure the right balance of macros.

o Make a shopping list of everything you're likely to need, and then take some time to sort out your kitchen cupboards. This would be a good time to get rid of anything that might derail your programme, or if that's not an option for the rest of the household, move it to a separate cupboard, so that it's out of your eyeline.

3. **Get creative with recipes**

o I've suggested plenty of meal ideas that you can adapt to suit your preferences, but I haven't provided recipes. There are so many great ones online – just Google the name of the dish and choose one that suits you!

o **Don't worry if you don't like any of the suggested meals.** The ideas set out in the table are simply suggestions to give you a bit of inspiration and provide examples of different ways to achieve the correct balance of macronutrients. It's absolutely fine if you prefer to use your own recipes and favourite meals. I'd recommend that you carefully read the advice on proteins, fats and carbohydrates in this chapter and draw on the information in the food tables to tweak your recipes to fit the principles of the programme.

YOUR DAILY MEAL & HYDRATION SCHEDULE	
MORNING	
Action	**Meal suggestions**
On waking	Drink a glass of water
Breakfast	2 eggs or tofu scrambled on wholemeal or rye toast
	2 poached eggs with ½ avocado and wilted spinach
	2 boiled eggs with asparagus tips
	Sweet potato and egg or tofu hash with roasted tomatoes
	Egg and mushroom muffins with wilted spinach
	30g overnight oats with 2 tablespoons pumpkin seeds, sunflower seeds or ground flaxseed, with 100g fresh fruit and natural or soya yogurt
	30g low-sugar granola or muesli with fruit and seeds, as above with authentic Greek yogurt (9g protein per 100g) or soya yogurt
	Wholemeal or rye toast with unsweetened peanut butter, cottage cheese or low-sugar baked beans
	Avocado and cottage cheese on wholemeal toast
	Chia seed pudding with Greek or soya yogurt and blueberries. Try grating in some orange zest or add a vanilla pod for extra flavour.

YOUR DAILY MEAL & HYDRATION SCHEDULE

MORNING

Action	Meal suggestions
Breakfast (continued)	Stewed apple or pear with 35g pumpkin and sunflower seeds and natural or soya yogurt
	Smoothie with 20g porridge oats, 1 tablespoon unsweetened almond or cashew butter, 2 handfuls raspberries or blueberries, 1 handful baby spinach, 1 tablespoon ground flaxseed, 1 tablespoon chia seeds, 250ml dairy or plant milk
	Porridge made with 30g oats; 1 tablespoon peanut, cashew or almond butter; 1 tablespoon ground flaxseed, 100g chopped apple or berries, 200ml dairy or plant milk
Mid-morning	Drink a glass of water
Breakfast tip	Soaking oats or seeds in milk, yogurt or water overnight makes them easier to digest and saves you time in the morning. Just add liquid before bed, and wake up to a quick, nutritious breakfast – no cooking required! Remember that yogurt or milk alone isn't always enough for protein, but combining them with seeds ensures a balanced start to your day.

DAYTIME	
Action	**Meal suggestions**
Before lunch	Drink a glass of water
Lunch	Make your own poke bowl with brown rice or quinoa; chicken, salmon, mackerel or tofu; and a combination of grated courgette/zucchini and carrots, shredded cabbage or sauerkraut, chopped cucumber, a sprinkle of pine nuts, fresh coriander/cilantro, a dash of soy sauce and sesame oil. Adapt the vegetable selection to your taste.
	Sardines, smoked tofu or roasted mushrooms on wholemeal toast. Liven it up a bit by spreading houmous or tzatziki on the bread before adding the sardines. Top with chopped olives, thinly sliced cherry tomatoes and a sprinkle of oregano.
	Mashed avocado on rye bread with a poached egg or sliced mushroom, and mixed leaves on the side
	Chicken, lentil and vegetable soup, or chickpea/garbanzo bean, sweet potato and lentil soup, to provide a double-whammy of protein to keep you going. Opt for a wholemeal roll if you want bread with it.
	Courgette/zucchini frittata with feta, garlic and mint, with a tomato and onion salad

DAYTIME

Action	Meal suggestions
Lunch (continued)	Sandwich suggestions: - Grilled chicken and avocado, with lettuce and tomato - Tuna mixed with Greek yogurt instead of mayonnaise, chopped celery and spinach leaves - Crushed falafel and houmous with rocket/arugula and cucumber - Smoked salmon and cream cheese with cucumber - Ham hock and egg mayonnaise with watercress - Smoked tempeh slices with soy sauce, mashed avocado, a squeeze of lime, spinach leaves and cucumber NB: please use wholemeal or rye bread
	Mixed salad with 2 eggs, chicken, tuna, salmon, crispy tofu, edamame beans or chickpeas/garbanzo beans. Use a base of green salad leaves, such as baby spinach, rocket/arugula, lamb's lettuce or curly kale. Add at least two more vegetables: cherry tomatoes, roasted peppers, mushrooms, beetroot, grated carrot, artichoke hearts, cucumber, celery, sugar snaps/sugar snap peas, green beans, baby corn or anything else you like. Make your own vinaigrette or yogurt-based dressing. It's much nicer and less processed than anything you can buy.
After lunch	If you want something sweet straight after lunch, have an apple, pear or satsuma.

DAYTIME	
Action	**Meal suggestions**
Lunchtime tips	Remember to aim for a fist-sized portion of both protein and starch to make up half your meal, and complete it with two portions of vegetables. That might require a bit of lateral thinking with a sandwich, but the principle remains the same. If you're buying a ready-made lunch, make sure that it contains a decent portion of protein. This is usually the most expensive ingredient, so outlets can often skimp on that part, which leaves you open to a mid-afternoon energy slump.
Mid-afternoon	Drink a glass of water

LATE AFTERNOON & EVENING	
Action	**Meal suggestions**
Before you leave work or log off for the day	Drink a glass of water
Before dinner	Drink a glass of water

LATE AFTERNOON & EVENING

Action	Meal suggestions
Dinner	Grilled salmon with brown rice, broccoli and green beans
	Shepherd's pie with half meat and half lentils (or all lentils), topped with sweet potato mash and served with mixed vegetables
	Roast chicken, beef or lamb, with new potatoes in their skins, peas, carrots and cauliflower
	Cod roasted with cherry tomatoes, leeks, fennel, olives and basil, served with quinoa
	Roasted vegetables, e.g. butternut squash, carrots, parsnips, red onion, bell peppers, courgette/zucchini, served with quinoa
	Classic spaghetti Bolognese, or lentil and mushroom Bolognese, with wholewheat pasta and a green salad
	Stir-fry with chicken, tofu or prawns. Add beansprouts, shredded cabbage, broccoli florets, mushrooms, onion, ginger and garlic. Season with soy sauce. Serve with wholewheat noodles or brown rice.
	Chilli con carne or chilli with black beans, kidney beans and lentils. Serve with brown rice, wholemeal tortilla or a jacket potato.
	Carrot and lentil dal, served with wilted spinach and crispy garlic

LATE AFTERNOON & EVENING

Action	Meal suggestions
Dinner (continued)	Goat's cheese and mushroom omelette with fresh thyme and grilled tomatoes and wilted spinach, or a mixed leaf salad, with a homemade vinaigrette
After dinner	Finish off the meal with a cup of herbal tea: peppermint, liquorice, fennel or rooibos/redbush with vanilla all work well after food, and can help to satisfy any cravings for sweet things.
Dinnertime tips	Make rice or quinoa more interesting by cooking it with a stock cube and stirring in chopped herbs after cooking, e.g. basil, coriander/cilantro or tarragon, then adding a squeeze of lemon. Remember to manage your portions, so that the starch is only a quarter of the overall meal. It's very common for rice or pasta to take over the plate, which simply isn't necessary.

Energy Boost FAQs

1. **What sort of refined carbohydrates and sugary foods do I need to avoid?**
   Swapping to wholemeal bread, brown rice and wholewheat pasta will eliminate a lot of refined carbs straight away. Opt for oat- or bran-based cereals, as these are usually made with complex carbohydrates. Steer clear of cakes, cookies and other baked products, and avoid confectionery, such as chocolate or other sweet treats. It's also important not to be drinking your sugar: a lot of soft drinks can be very high in sugar (see point 8).

2. **Why can I only eat two portions of fruit each day?**
   There are lots of benefits to eating fruit, because it's full of vitamins and minerals. However, it does also contain large amounts of fruit sugar, which can affect your blood sugar balance if you're eating it in large quantities, and this may impact your energy levels. Excessive levels of fruit can also be a common culprit in bloating and digestive discomfort. There is a tendency to skew our 5-a-day fruit and vegetables toward fruit because it's tastier, but we'd actually benefit far more from increasing our vegetables. This is why I recommend at least four portions of vegetables each day.

3. **I don't usually eat breakfast. Is that a problem?**
   If you're experiencing low energy and fatigue, then skipping breakfast may well be a problem. If you want to achieve the full benefit of the 14-day programme, I'd advise you to stick with the three-meal-a-day approach. It's fine to have just a small breakfast, if you find it hard to eat in the morning. Options could include a slice of wholemeal toast with nut butter, or a small portion of stewed apple with mixed seeds.

4. **I don't eat starchy carbs with my evening meal. Do I need to start?**
   If you tend to avoid starchy foods such as rice, pasta or potatoes in the evening, that's perfectly fine. You might do this because they feel too heavy on digestion in the evening, or because you're watching your weight. If so, you can adjust the balance by ensuring that protein still makes up a quarter of your meal, while replacing the starchy option with an extra portion of vegetables, so that vegetables make up three-quarters of the meal.

   If you have a physically demanding job and feel very tired in the evening, you may benefit from incorporating some extra starch during the day. In this case, it's advisable to include starchy foods such as rice or potatoes at lunchtime to help fuel your afternoon energy.

5. **Why can't I have a healthy snack?**
   The reason that I've removed snacks is because of the challenges we face with our metabolism as we transition through the menopause. Our metabolic rate slows down, and weight gain can be a common problem. If you're in the habit of grazing throughout the day, you will have trained your body to expect a constant supply of food. If you have three nutritious meals a day and leave proper gaps between eating, this will support your digestion and stabilize your blood sugar. It may take a bit of getting used to, but your body will adapt to this, so that it starts to process food as energy, instead of storing it as fat.

   If your schedule is completely erratic and you have no control over when you can eat, then opt for a balanced protein–fibre snack such as six or seven raw almonds with an apple, or some carrot sticks with a 50g portion of houmous.

However, ideally, for these two weeks, you should stick with three meals a day and no snacks. This is how you'll derive the most benefit.

6. **How much water should I be drinking in the programme?**
The schedule includes some reminders for drinking water throughout the day to get you started. However, our hydration requirements are highly individual, so you may need more than this. See page 77 for more advice on optimal hydration.

7. **Why can I only have two caffeinated drinks each day?**
Caffeine can have a big impact on our energy levels and is a major sleep disruptor. A small amount of caffeine every day is fine for most people, but if you consistently rely on it to keep you going throughout the day, that suggests an underlying energy issue that needs addressing. Reducing it to a moderate amount (or avoiding it altogether, if you can manage that) can make a big difference to the quality of your sleep and your overall energy levels. You can find out more about the caffeine content of different products on pages 215–17.

Caffeinated drinks	Caffeine-free alternatives
Coffee	Decaffeinated coffee (opt for a chemical-free one)
Black tea, white tea, green tea, jasmine tea	Rooibos/redbush tea
Colas	Herbal teas, such as peppermint, camomile, lemongrass or fennel
Carbonated energy drinks	Fruit teas
	Sugar-free sodas made with sparkling water and a dash of fruit juice

8. **What soft drinks can I have?**

   A lot of soft drinks can be quite sugary. I'd recommend avoiding carbonated drinks such as cola or lemonade, as well as fruit juices and smoothies, which are often high in sugar. Water or sparkling water are the best choices.

   I often enjoy sparkling water with lime cordial when I'm at a bar. Tonic water is another great option for a non-alcoholic soft drink, and flavoured varieties such as elderflower tonic can be very refreshing. A newer option to consider are the cans of sparkling water with no added sugar, featuring small amounts of fruit juice for a hint of flavour. Be sure to check the label to ensure they remain relatively low in sugar (4g of sugar is about a teaspoon, to help you keep on track).

9. **Will I lose weight on this programme?**

   The Energy Boost programme is not designed to be a weight-loss diet. However, you may well find that you lose a few pounds, simply because you're avoiding many of the common culprits in weight-gain, such as sugary treats, alcohol and excessive portions. As your energy improves, you may also be more inclined to exercise, which would improve muscle tone and body shape.

10. **Can I have dessert?**

    During the 14-day period, desserts are best avoided, because of the sugar levels involved. You could have a piece of fruit after lunch, provided that doesn't make you feel bloated, which can sometimes happen if you eat fruit after a meal. In the evening, I'd suggest rounding off with a cup of herbal tea, rather than a sugary dessert, if you want to achieve the full effect of the programme.

After the programme

Once you reach the end of your 14-day programme, you should already have observed some improvements in your strength and stamina. It's time to score your symptoms again.

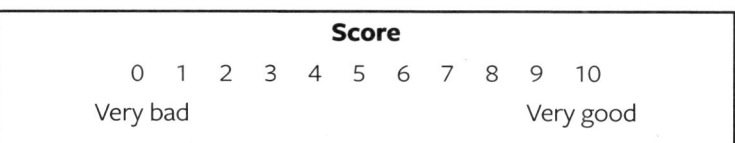

Score

| 0 | 1 | 2 | 3 | 4 | 5 | 6 | 7 | 8 | 9 | 10 |

Very bad   Very good

Record your score out of 10 in your notebook for each of these areas that can be affected by fatigue: physical energy, strength, stamina, memory, concentration, mental clarity. Once you've done this, you can compare it to the scores you gave yourself before you started. What changes have you noticed?

Energy Action Plan – my next steps

Over the course of the past two weeks, you've got into the habit of balancing your macronutrients more carefully, which will have made a difference in a number of ways. Take a moment to reflect on the changes you've made and which of them you feel have been most beneficial to you.

Areas to consider

- Have you benefited from eating protein more regularly?
- Are you less reliant on caffeine for energy?
- Has avoiding alcohol improved your quality of sleep?
- Do you feel better without eating sugary treats and snacks?

- How have you coped with having three sustaining meals a day, instead of constant grazing? What difference has it made?
- Did you find that complex carbohydrates kept you going for longer?
- How did you get on with maintaining your hydration levels?
- How easy or difficult did you find these changes?
- Which of these changes do you feel has made the most difference for you?

Record your conclusions in your notebook and use it as an opportunity to build on the progress you've made so far. The more consistently you commit to these changes, the more improvement you are likely to see.

Focus on these three questions to create your SMART objectives:

1. What will I do?
2. How will I do it?
3. When will I do it by?

WHERE DO I GO FROM HERE?

To continue benefiting from the improvements in your health and wellbeing, it's important to maintain a balanced approach to macronutrients and hydration, ensuring this becomes a natural part of your meal planning.

Now that you've seen the impact a few dietary adjustments can have, I recommend adopting the **80:20 rule**. This means aiming for **nutrient-dense, balanced meals at least 80 per cent of the time**, while allowing **20 per cent for flexibility**, so you can enjoy the occasional treat or indulgence without guilt. It's about long-term balance, not perfection!

Here's some guidance to support you in maintaining your progress. You may find it helpful to incorporate some of the reflections you've noted down, helping you keep on track as you progress through The Happy Menopause Energy Clinic.

After the programme: maintenance tips

1. Every meal should feature a combination of protein and fibre.
2. Always respect the quadrant proportions of protein, complex carbs and two vegetables at lunch and dinner when plating up or choosing a meal at a restaurant.
3. Continue to monitor your hydration, so you maintain the good habits you've put in place.
4. Your 5-a-day ratio should be 4 veg:1 fruit, or if you want more fruit, make it 5 veg:2 fruits.
5. Eat fruit, don't drink it!
6. Continue to limit your caffeine intake to a maximum of two caffeinated drinks per day or less, if you feel better without it.
7. It's fine to have a moderate amount of alcohol from time to time. Make sure this doesn't start to creep up over the course of the week. A helpful approach is to aim for at least four **consecutive** alcohol-free days each week, building on the progress you've made in the past fortnight.
8. The occasional sugary indulgence or dessert is fine, as long as it's not too often. Remember that a treat is something that is out of the ordinary, not something you have every day!

Now that you've mastered the basics, it's time to fine-tune your approach to boost your energy to 10/10. In the next chapter, you'll have another virtual consultation with The Happy Menopause Energy Clinic. This section features a series of short quizzes designed to help you pinpoint your personal energy weak points. Once you've identified these, you can follow tailored advice to address these issues by integrating the recommended diet and lifestyle changes for lasting results.

STEP 4

DISCOVER TARGETED SOLUTIONS FOR MICRONUTRIENT IMBALANCES

In the previous chapter, you focused on getting the energy basics of your diet right with the correct macronutrient (i.e. protein, fat and carbohydrate) and fluid balance. I hope that you're already feeling the benefits of the adjustments you've made over the past 14 days. Now it's time to explore some of the more complex factors that could be playing a part in your fatigue. In this stage of The Happy Menopause Energy Clinic, we'll examine potential micronutrient and functional imbalances.

THE HAPPY MENOPAUSE ENERGY QUIZ

The first section in this chapter is a series of energy quizzes, which act as a form of triage to help you identify the potential underlying factors in your lack of energy. In my real-world clinic, this is where we'd be running some functional tests. I've devised the quizzes as a virtual way of exploring these areas.

You'll need to complete each quiz and then move on to the section or sections that are the most relevant to you, depending on your results.

Get your notebook ready, as there will be plenty of opportunities for reflection! Once you've read through each section, you'll need to note down your action points, based on what you've learned.

How do the quizzes work?

The symptoms in each box correspond to a specific issue that can commonly cause fatigue. The shaded area highlights the more frequent symptoms, although all the symptoms listed could be associated with that particular issue.

Count up the various symptoms that you're experiencing in each box to identify what could be affecting your energy levels. Then follow the instructions beneath each quiz to learn your score and to discover the potential underlying cause of your symptoms.

You may find that you score highly in more than one quiz, which is not unusual. Fatigue often arises from multiple contributory factors. Simply read the relevant sections and apply the advice provided. You can take a step-by-step approach or implement all the recommended changes at once, whichever suits you best.

QUIZ 1

Do you experience energy highs and lows?

Do you struggle to lose abdominal fat?

Do you ever feel dizzy or irritable if you don't eat?

Do you crave sugary foods or carbohydrate?

Do you rely on caffeine or sugar to keep you going?

Do you leave long gaps between meals?

Do you feel lightheaded or dizzy if you stand up quickly?

Do you find it difficult to concentrate?

Quiz 1: What's my score?

If you experience three or more of these symptoms, including any two from the shaded section, this is likely to indicate a blood sugar imbalance. This is one of the most common culprits in energy issues and a fundamental area to address to improve your physical and mental vitality. Go to page 113 to learn more about blood sugar and discover practical steps to help keep it in balance.

QUIZ 2

Do you feel persistent tiredness unrelieved by rest?

Have you gained weight?

Is your hair thinning?

Do you feel the cold?

Do you struggle with constipation?

Do you feel anxious or low?

Do you feel less alert and focused?

Are you unusually forgetful?

Are your nails brittle?

Do you have muscle aches or cramps?

Do you find it hard to lose weight, even if you're really strict with yourself?

Do you have dry skin?

Quiz 2: What's my score?

If you experience five or more of these symptoms (including at least two of the shaded symptoms) on a regular basis, this may indicate an underactive thyroid. Go to page 126 to learn more about the thyroid, how it might affect your energy levels and what action you should take.

QUIZ 3

Do you lack strength and stamina, and feel physically weak?

Do you get regular headaches?

Do you experience palpitations?

Do you have shortness of breath?

Is your skin paler than usual?

Do you have thinning hair?

Are you feeling unusually anxious?

Are you a vegan or following a mainly plant-based diet?

Do you have a sore tongue?

Do you struggle to concentrate?

Do you experience heavy periods or flooding?

Have you got tinnitus?

Do you bruise easily?

Quiz 3: What's my score?

If you experience five or more of these symptoms (including at least three of the shaded symptoms) on a regular basis, it's possible that iron deficiency anaemia is the cause. Go to page 147 to learn more about the role of iron in the energy production process and how you can optimize your iron levels.

QUIZ 4

Do you feel constantly tired?

Are you a vegan or following a mainly plant-based diet?

Do you struggle to focus and concentrate?

Are you experiencing low mood?

Does your brain feel confused and "foggy"?

Do you struggle with memory issues?

Do you experience clumsiness or loss of coordination

Do you feel breathless?

Do you get regular pins and needles?

Do you struggle with indigestion?

Quiz 4: What's my score?

If you experience five or more of these symptoms (including at least four of the shaded symptoms), it's worth exploring whether low levels of vitamin B12 might be the problem. Go to page 160 to learn about vitamin B12, why it's important for your energy levels and how to address a suspected deficiency.

QUIZ 5

Are you tired all the time?

Do you feel as if you're only operating on sheer willpower?

Are you unusually anxious or irritable?

Do you struggle to switch off?

Do your muscles or joints ache?

Are you constipated?

Do you find it hard to go to sleep?

Do you have restless legs?

Are you finding it harder than usual to manage stress?

Quiz 5: What's my score?

If you experience five or more of these symptoms (including at least three of the shaded symptoms), it's possible that low levels of magnesium are the problem. Go to page 171 to learn about magnesium, why it might be affecting your energy levels and what you can do about it.

QUIZ 6

Do you have bone pain, back pain or muscle weakness?

Do you have repeated colds or infections?

Do you have unexplained fatigue?

Do you suffer with Seasonal Affective Disorder?

Do you suffer from low mood or depression?

Are your wounds slow to heal?

Do you struggle with insomnia?

Do you have general aches and pains?

Quiz 6: What's my score?

If you experience four or more of these symptoms (including at least two of the shaded symptoms), you might be suffering from a vitamin D deficiency. Go to page 181 to learn about vitamin D, the role it plays in your energy levels and how to address a suspected deficiency.

QUIZ 7

Do you feel tired or lethargic, especially after eating?

Do you experience bloating, wind or abdominal pain?

Have you started to suffer from constipation, diarrhoea or urgency?

Do you have skin rashes or issues with eczema or dermatitis?

Are you prone to headaches?

Do you have muscle or joint pain?

Do you feel nauseous?

Do you have sinusitis, rhinitis or post-nasal drip?

Do you feel tired all the time?

Quiz 7: What's my score?

Any of the symptoms in this box may indicate a food sensitivity, although the shaded ones are more characteristic of an issue. You don't need to experience multiple symptoms to suspect a potential problem. If your doctor has ruled out any medical conditions or functional imbalances related to any of these symptoms, and you're still struggling with one or more of them, it's worth exploring the possibility of a food sensitivity. Turn to page 191 to learn more about this complex topic and discover the best ways to address it.

Next steps

Now that you've completed the quiz and tallied your results, it's time to delve into the possible root causes of your tiredness. Each section below corresponds to one of the quizzes above. Review these sections to identify the one(s) most relevant to you. You'll find a comprehensive guide for each issue, complete with detailed diet and lifestyle advice to help you take the next steps in your Energy Action Plan. There'll be an opportunity to reflect on each section and to make a note of anything that resonates with you.

YOUR GUIDE TO BLOOD SUGAR BALANCE

If you scored highly in Quiz 1, this is the section for you!

In my nutrition clinic, blood sugar balance is a crucial first step whatever I've been consulted about, because it can impact the body in so many positive ways. If you've carefully followed the 14-Day Energy Boost Programme in Step 3, you may already be well on the way to managing your blood sugar effectively without realizing it, and I hope you've started to notice a tangible difference.

How does blood sugar affect my energy levels?

The key word here is *balance*. It's not about demonizing sugar. Glucose is a quick-and-easy source of energy for the body. It's also the primary source of energy for the brain, ensuring optimal function of the neurotransmitters that keep it firing on all cylinders.

Too little glucose in the blood and you will quickly feel tired, irritable, shaky and find it difficult to concentrate or be creative and productive. Too much glucose in the blood can affect mood, memory and focus, due to the impact of excess sugar on the neural pathways.

If you have the right balance of blood glucose, you'll benefit from sustained physical and mental energy, and will feel so much better, stronger and sharper.

A blood sugar imbalance can also significantly impact mitochondrial function, interfering with the production of energy. Maintaining blood sugar balance supports the efficient utilization of glucose to produce ATP molecules, the body's energy storage units. When blood sugar levels are either too high or too low, mitochondrial efficiency is reduced, leading to decreased ATP production and increased oxidative stress which can damage your mitochondrial DNA. Chronic blood sugar imbalances can accelerate mitochondrial ageing, impairing their ability to regenerate and maintain optimal function.

How the body regulates blood sugar

Our very clever body is programmed to keep everything in balance so that we don't need to worry about it. It has all manner of ingenious systems that address any imbalances before you even become aware of them, through a regulatory process called homeostasis.

Homeostasis will regulate blood sugar, body temperature, fluid balance, blood pressure, the pH (acid–alkaline) balance, oxygen levels and anything else that is out of balance. The body has its own detox systems too.

We don't need to be spending a fortune on miracle detox powders, drinking vinegar or following radical regimes to keep in balance. That simply won't help. All we need to do is give our body the tools to do the job, and it will take care of everything for us, so that you don't have to think about it.

The body is programmed to keep levels of sugar in the blood within a certain range. If levels go significantly above or below this range, it will take prompt action, because both high blood sugar and low blood sugar can be very disruptive to a whole range of systems in the body.

A blood sugar spike will prompt the pancreas to release insulin to redress the balance. Insulin's job is to scoop the sugar out of the blood and send it off to the liver to be stored as glycogen. This is an energy store that the body can draw on as required.

If you've been consuming a lot of sugar and the glycogen stores are already full, any excess sugar will be stored as fat cells. This is why excessive levels of sugar and carbohydrate are such a common cause of weight gain.

The blood sugar seesaw

A blood sugar spike will be followed by a blood sugar crash – basically, what goes up, must come down! The emergency response of insulin won't precisely restore blood sugar levels to the required range, it simply hoovers up the whole lot. In a short space of time, your blood sugar will crash and this is when you'll experience so many of the symptoms listed in the Quiz 1.

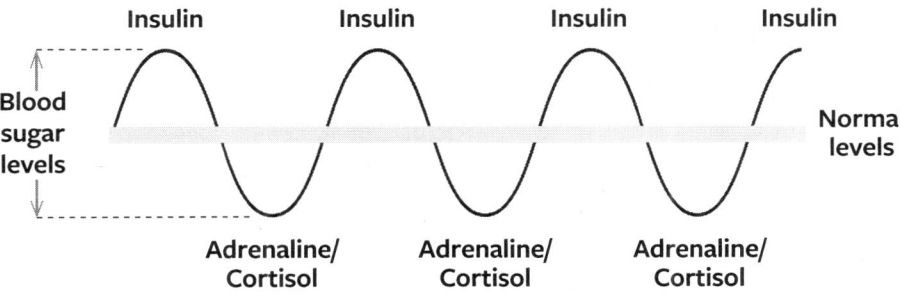

Low blood sugar triggers an immediate hormonal response, and this is where the two principal stress hormones, adrenaline and cortisol, will come into play.

It's dangerous not to have enough sugar in the blood – it's our primary source of energy – so this will trigger a stress response in the body, activating our primeval fight-or-flight response. We're still genetically programmed for conditions 10,000 years ago and this emergency response is designed to protect us against imminent physical danger, such as a sabre-toothed tiger or other predator. As lack of energy affects our ability to fight or to flee, the body needs to take prompt action.

Adrenaline will increase the heart rate; this may cause sweating, nervousness, irritability and headaches. Together with cortisol, adrenaline regulates blood glucose levels by encouraging the liver to re-release the sugar stores. Cortisol will also trigger urgent cravings for sugary food or refined carbohydrate to redress the balance.

As a result, there's a dual effect, where the liver releases the sugar stores, and you reach for a quick sugary fix. In the short term, you'll feel better.

The problem, however, is that instead of going back to the optimum range for blood sugar balance, the body's two-pronged approach will lead to another blood sugar spike. This will cause the whole process to start again, so that these highs and lows of blood sugar will be the background to your day, constantly draining your physical and mental energy.

Typical signs of a blood sugar imbalance

- Fatigue
- Energy highs and lows
- Poor concentration and memory
- Brain fog
- Dizziness
- Insomnia

- Headaches
- Anxiety
- Irritability
- Difficulty losing weight
- Abdominal fat
- Pre-menstrual syndrome (PMS)
- Craving for sugary food or carbs

Why might the menopause affect my blood sugar balance?

The decline in oestrogen as we transition through menopause can affect insulin sensitivity, which is why there is an increased risk of diabetes post-menopause. Insulin sensitivity is the way in which our body cells respond to insulin in order to balance blood sugar effectively.

If the cells become less sensitive to insulin, increasingly higher levels are required to balance the blood sugar. Over a long period of time, this may lead to a state of insulin resistance, which is a prediabetic state in which the body stops responding to insulin altogether. It's wise to pre-empt this possibility by maintaining blood sugar balance as a matter of course.

A little help from cinnamon

Cinnamon has natural properties that balance blood sugar. Sprinkling a spoonful over your morning cereal or porridge instead of sugar adds flavour and supports sustained energy levels.

However, it's also worth asking the reverse: how does blood sugar balance affect my menopause? This is something I cover extensively in my book *The Happy Menopause: Smart Nutrition to Help You Flourish*, which is a symptom-by-symptom guide to managing your menopause with nutrition. It includes a whole chapter dedicated to blood sugar balance, which you may find helpful if you're experiencing other symptoms beyond low energy or fatigue.

A blood sugar imbalance can make other symptoms much worse. For example, the increase in stress hormones adrenaline and cortisol will exacerbate menopause symptoms (see page 244) and make you more likely to gain weight and/or find it difficult to lose weight. A blood sugar imbalance is also a frequent cause of disturbed sleep or insomnia (see page 259).

If you're in perimenopause and still having periods (even if they're erratic), excessive levels of adrenaline can also interfere with the action of progesterone in the second half of your cycle. This could exacerbate psychological and emotional symptoms before your period, increase PMS and cause the common issue of "feeling hormonal".

Typical causes of a blood sugar imbalance

- Excessive consumption of sugary foods and refined carbohydrate
- Too many sugary drinks
- Disruptive impact of caffeine and alcohol on the insulin response
- Lack of dietary fibre
- Low levels of protein in the diet
- Long gaps between meals
- Menopausal hormone changes

Testing your blood sugar

If you're concerned about your blood glucose levels, you should consult your doctor, who would want to rule out any issues with insulin resistance, or type 1 or type 2 diabetes that may be contributing to your fatigue.

See page 26 to understand more about the different tests your doctor may advise. It's important to note that these tests would be specifically targeting diabetes, which is a chronic health condition that requires medical support. A blood sugar imbalance is not the same thing. If your test results are normal and you display a number of the symptoms in Quiz 1, it is very likely that you will still benefit significantly from focusing on blood sugar balance.

HOW TO BALANCE BLOOD SUGAR THROUGH DIET

Maintaining stable blood sugar levels requires a two-pronged approach:

1. Limit food or drinks that will cause a blood sugar spike and activate or disrupt the insulin response.

2. Focus on food or drinks that provide or support a slow release of energy into the body to keep the appropriate blood sugar balance.

FOODS TO REDUCE FOR BALANCED BLOOD SUGAR

Food type	Examples
Refined carbohydrate	White bread, white rice, white pasta, white noodles, white flour, refined sugar, cakes, cookies, baked goods, refined breakfast cereals
Sugary products	Chocolate, sweets or candy, fruit yogurts, undiluted fruit juice, ice cream, prepared sauces and certain condiments, sodas, jam, honey
Stimulants	Alcohol; caffeinated drinks, e.g. tea, green tea, coffee, cola, energy drinks; nicotine

Excessive levels of sugary foods and refined carbohydrate will inevitably cause the blood sugar to spike. Stimulants interfere with the insulin response in a different way, but the overall effect will disrupt blood sugar balance, so they need to be taken just as seriously.

Keeping these foods or drinks to a minimum and prioritizing the foods in the table on page 122 is the simplest way to balance your blood sugar and ensure sustained energy levels.

Understand sugar labelling

Be aware of hidden sugar. A surprising number of everyday foods contain more sugar than you might expect. Common culprits include fruit yogurt, certain breakfast cereals, fruit juice and some pasta sauces.

Sugar is a natural component of carbohydrate (see page 63), so it's always going to feature on the label of something that includes carbohydrate, such as bread or pasta. That's quite normal and you don't need to be too concerned about it. You'll only find zero sugar if you're buying a product that doesn't contain carbohydrate at all, such as fresh meat or fish.

However, if the product contains more than 10g of sugar per portion, that's heading toward quite a lot of added sugar. It would be advisable to look for a product that's lower in sugar or consume a smaller portion, to keep the impact to a minimum.

Check the label

If you want to be sugar savvy, check the label. 4g of sugar is about a teaspoon, so you can do the maths. For example, if a product contains 16g of sugar per serving (not per 100g, which is often very different), that will add up to 4 teaspoons of sugar.

Moderate caffeine & alcohol intake

Don't panic! I'm not suggesting that you have to give up tea, coffee or alcohol altogether. It's all about moderation.

If you're having more than 2–3 cups of tea or coffee every day, this is likely to affect your blood sugar. Identify the important ones and cut out the rest or swap them for caffeine-free alternatives.

For example, the first tea or coffee of the day may be non-negotiable. That's fine, so long as your breakfast is nicely balanced with protein and fibre, and you're not also having a large glass of orange juice, a croissant and jam, or a sugary cereal at the same time. That would be a fast route to a blood sugar spike before you've even left the house!

Some alcoholic drinks can give a double-whammy of sugar and stimulant. While it's wise to moderate your alcohol consumption in order to maintain blood sugar balance, avoiding the more sugary options when you do have a drink would also be sensible. Beer, lager, cider, rosé wine and sparkling wines all tend to be pretty high in sugar. Opt for red wine, dry white wine, gin and tonic, or vodka and soda if you want to keep the sugar levels down.

The truth about green tea

It may be a surprise to learn that green tea contains roughly the same amount of caffeine as black tea. It comes from the same plant.

FOODS TO PRIORITIZE FOR BALANCED BLOOD SUGAR

Food type	Examples
Complex carbohydrate (fibre)	Wholegrain foods, e.g. wholemeal bread, brown rice, wholegrain pasta; oats, sweet potato, pulses, vegetables, fruits with an edible skin
Protein	Meat, fish, eggs, dairy products, soya bean, tofu, lentils, chickpeas/garbanzo beans, houmous, beans, quinoa, nuts and seeds
Drinks	Water, sparkling water, herbal teas, caffeine-free teas, e.g. rooibos/redbush, water-processed decaffeinated coffee (to limit the chemicals), diluted fruit juice ($\frac{1}{3}$ juice to $\frac{2}{3}$ water), vegetable juices

Complex carbohydrate is rich in fibre. The body burns through it much more slowly than refined or simple carbohydrates or sugars. It provides a sustained source of energy which will keep you going for longer.

Protein is hard to digest, so it slows down the release of the carbohydrate into the blood, maintaining a stable blood sugar balance until your next meal.

The simplest way to balance blood sugar is to eat a combination of protein and fibre with every meal and every snack.

Follow the quadrant approach set out in Step 3 (see the plate diagram, page 69) to ensure that you're managing your portions correctly and maintaining the appropriate balance of macronutrients to keep your blood sugar in good order.

EXAMPLES OF BLOOD SUGAR-BALANCING MEALS*

Breakfast	Lunch	Dinner	Snacks
Poached egg or scrambled tofu with wilted spinach and avocado	A wholemeal sandwich with tuna, watercress and cucumber	Grilled chicken with teriyaki glaze, brown rice, broccoli and green beans	A small slice of rye bread with unsweetened peanut butter or houmous
Overnight oats in Greek yogurt with blueberries and 2 tablespoons pumpkin or sunflower seeds	A salmon or falafel poke bowl with mixed vegetables, a drizzle of tahini and sesame seeds	Vegetable chilli served with quinoa, topped with sliced avocado, coriander/cilantro and natural yogurt	7–8 raw unsalted almonds with an apple
Baked beans or almond butter with sesame seeds on wholemeal toast	Grilled chicken or halloumi with roasted sweet potato, mixed greens and a lemon and olive oil dressing	A bell pepper stuffed with quinoa, black beans, diced tomato and grated cheese	An energy ball, made by blending dates, almonds, oats, a touch of honey, and cacao powder; roll into bite-sized balls and refrigerate

* Refer to page 69 for advice on portions. Simple recipes for any of these dishes are easily available online.

CASE STUDY: A solution for sugar dependency – Andrea's story

Andrea, 52, came to my clinic worried about her weight and frustrated by her lack of energy and irritability. At our initial consultation, she admitted to having a sweet tooth and struggling to reduce the sugar in her diet. She relied on sugary treats to keep her going, particularly in the afternoons when she often experienced a severe energy crash.

A review of her food diary and health questionnaire revealed clear signs of blood sugar imbalance. Her diet was high in starch and sugar, with limited protein and very little fibre. Once I explained how blood sugar works and how protein can reduce sugar cravings and improve satiety, Andrea was relieved to know there was a solution.

Over several months, we worked together to tackle her sugar dependency – no small feat, as sugar can be highly addictive. By the end of the process, Andrea had mastered balancing her blood sugar, prioritizing protein and increasing her fibre intake. She'd dropped a dress size and rediscovered her energy and motivation!

Easy ways to maintain blood sugar balance

- Avoid sugary foods and confectionery.
- Swap white foods (e.g. white bread, white rice, white pasta) for brown foods, such as wholemeal bread, brown rice, wholegrain pasta.
- Aim for three sustaining meals per day with no snacks in between. You should only require a snack if there's an unusually long gap between your meals.
- Eat more vegetables: aim for five portions of vegetables every day.
- Add protein to your morning cereal with 2 tablespoons of mixed seeds or chopped nuts.

- Add lentils or beans to vegetable soups, or stir in some ground flaxseed to boost the protein content.
- Make sure you have a balanced snack in your bag, if you're going to be out and about and likely to miss a meal.
- Don't drink your sugar: opt for sparkling water with a dash of cordial; dilute your fruit juices; avoid sugary sodas.
- Manage your caffeine intake: if the breakfast coffee is non-negotiable, make sure the rest of the meal is designed to balance blood sugar.
- Moderate your alcohol intake. When you do drink alcohol, avoid the obviously sugary options.

Energy Action Plan – my next steps

What three things can you do to balance your blood sugar? Do you need to eat more protein? Are you consuming a lot of hidden sugars or refined carbohydrates? Is the balance of your portions correct? Where might you be falling short?

It's time to take out your notebook again! Jot down anything that stood out to you in this section and create a commitment to tackling the issue head-on.

Focus on these three questions to create your SMART objectives:

1. What will I do?
2. How will I do it?
3. When will I do it by?

YOUR GUIDE TO THE THYROID GLAND

If you scored highly in Quiz 2 (see page 106), read on to learn more about the thyroid gland and how it could be impacting your energy levels.

The thyroid is a small, butterfly-shaped gland that sits in the neck, and every body cell relies on it for optimum function and energy metabolism. This is why the symptoms of thyroid dysfunction can be so many and varied, although low energy and fatigue are probably the most significant of these.

If your energy quiz ticked a lot of boxes for the common symptoms for hypothyroidism (underactive thyroid), then you'll probably be feeling pretty rough, and this is definitely an area worth exploring with your doctor. An underactive thyroid is a condition that can often go unrecognized for women in midlife: it's easy to assume that the menopause is at the root of the problem, because many of the symptoms of menopause are identical to those of an underactive thyroid.

Many of the women I see in my nutrition clinic blame their fatigue on their hectic life or their age, not realizing that it's not normal to feel tired all the time, or for fatigue to be unrelieved by rest, however old you are.

As human beings, we are very adaptable and adjust to a new normal very quickly, so many of us get used to putting up with debilitating symptoms on a daily basis. If this sounds familiar, then it's time to seek some help from a medical professional.

How does the thyroid work?

The thyroid is part of the endocrine system, a complex network of glands and hormones that control a whole series of functions across the body. It's managed by something called a negative feedback loop, which is a self-regulating system, allowing the body to produce thyroid hormones whenever they are required or to stop whenever the correct balance has been achieved.

A cascade of Hormones

Thyroid function relies on a precise chain reaction. It all starts in the brain, where the hypothalamus releases thyrotropin-releasing hormone (TRH). This signals the pituitary gland to produce thyroid-stimulating hormone (TSH).

TSH then prompts the thyroid to release thyroxine (T4), which is later converted into triiodothyronine (T3) – the active hormone responsible for most thyroid functions.

The main thing to remember? TSH → T4 → T3. This is where things often go wrong. If any step in this process falters, thyroid hormone levels can become imbalanced, which will directly impact your energy levels.

How does the thyroid affect my energy levels?

The intricate balance of hormones that supports healthy thyroid function is delicate, so it's not surprising that things can sometimes go awry. While other forms of thyroid dysfunction may also lead to fatigue, hypothyroidism (an underactive thyroid) is the condition most frequently linked to tiredness.

If you're not producing enough T4 or T3, the thyroid may struggle to effectively support mitochondrial production, efficiency and energy metabolism.

T4 acts as a storage hormone, which delivers T3, the active thyroid hormone, to our body cells. T3 plays a crucial role in energy metabolism within the cells, whatever the function of that cell. This is why, alongside severe fatigue, the symptoms of an underactive thyroid are so diverse, leaving you feeling pretty rotten.

How does the menopause affect my thyroid function?

Our risk of developing an underactive thyroid increases with age, and women are far more likely to experience this condition than men. Midlife can be particularly challenging for some women, as fluctuating hormones create a perfect storm of symptoms. Since oestrogen receptors are present throughout the body – including in the thyroid – it's no surprise that your thyroid gland might struggle during this phase of life. That's why it's important to monitor your symptoms and seek medical advice if you're concerned.

A drop in oestrogen won't directly cause an underactive thyroid if your thyroid function is normal. However, if you are on HRT and you are already taking levothyroxine to manage an underactive thyroid, it may be necessary for your doctor to review the dosage of your thyroid medication, as oral oestrogen can affect the levels of free T4 in the blood.

Many symptoms of an underactive thyroid can overlap with those of perimenopause and menopause, so it's essential to consult with your doctor before assuming it's just another menopause-related issue.

Typical signs of an underactive thyroid

- Fatigue
- Low energy
- Sensitivity to the cold
- Weight gain or difficulty losing weight
- Low mood
- Anxiety
- Poor memory and concentration
- Thinning hair
- Brittle nails
- Muscle aches or weakness
- Loss of libido
- Constipation
- Irregular or heavy periods

UNDERSTANDING YOUR TEST RESULTS

If you're experiencing any of these symptoms, the first port of call should be your doctor. They will give you a blood test to assess the status of your thyroid hormones and decide whether you would benefit from medication.

Thyroid-stimulating hormone (TSH)

As we have seen above, there are several different thyroid hormones, but the one your doctor is most likely to test as a first step is TSH. Although it may seem counter-intuitive, high levels of TSH, rather than low levels, are an indicator of an underactive thyroid.

Unfortunately, this doesn't always provide the full picture. If there is a problem with the conversion process for T4 or T3, your TSH levels may present as normal, despite there being an issue further down the cascade. This is why it's worth requesting that your T4 and T3 levels are also tested, and even your thyroid antibodies. These are proteins produced by the immune system that can mistakenly attack the thyroid, potentially leading to an autoimmune condition called Hashimoto's thyroiditis, which can trigger an underactive thyroid.

Thyroxine (T4)

Two measures may be used here: total T4 and free T4. Total T4 measures the total amount of inactive thyroid hormone in the blood. Free T4 is the amount of T4 that is available for use by the body because it hasn't already bonded to the proteins in the blood. This is why a free T4 test is usually more revealing.

Triiodothyronine (T3)

As with T4, a total T3 test will capture the total amount of T3 in the blood. A free T3 test will establish the amount of T3 that hasn't bonded to proteins in the blood and is available for use. A free T3 test would be preferable to allow for the full picture of your hormonal status.

Other thyroid hormone tests include reverse T3, thyroid peroxidase antibodies, thyroglobulin antibodies and thyroid-stimulating immunoglobulins. These would normally only be assessed if your doctor has referred you to an endocrinologist for specialist assessment.

Reference ranges

A reference range is a scale which reflects the upper and lower limits of normal for a functional test, statistically based on a broad group of healthy people. The reference ranges for TSH, T4 and T3 can be pretty broad, so it is worth assessing what your result means for *you*. It can be very frustrating to be told that your results are "normal", when you're feeling absolutely exhausted, and you know that something isn't right.

Check where you are on the scale of your test results. You have every right to see them, so don't be shy about asking. If you're at the upper or lower end of the range this may still be too high or too low for you, regardless of the statistics. Normal is not the same thing as optimal, and this might explain why you're feeling so dreadful. The table below indicates where your scores should ideally be, for TSH, free T4 and free T3.

Hormone	Standard reference range	Optimal reference range
TSH	0.4–4.0 mU/L	1.0–2.0 mU/L
Free thyroxine or free T4 (FT4)	10–22 pmol/L	12–20 pmol/L
Free T3 (FT3)	2.8–6.5 pmol/L	3.4–6.0 pmol/L

If your doctor says that your scores are normal, you may be suffering from a sub-clinical thyroid, where your hormone levels are not sufficiently out of range to be of medical concern, but you're showing early symptoms of hypothyroidism. This is where your diet and lifestyle could really make a difference. The next section provides detailed guidance on how to create a thyroid-friendly diet.

Potential causes of a sub-clinical underactive thyroid

- Poor diet
- Nutrient deficiencies
- Chronic stress
- Trauma, e.g. bereavement, surgery or an accident of some description
- Poor liver function

- Radiation treatment of the thyroid
- A thyroidectomy
- Undiagnosed Hashimoto's thyroiditis
- Low levels of vitamin D may affect thyroid function

A predominantly female issue

Women are about ten times more likely than men to suffer from an underactive thyroid.

HOW TO SUPPORT YOUR THYROID FUNCTION THROUGH DIET

As with every chain reaction in the body, certain nutrients act as a catalyst to activate and support the cascade of hormones. If you're low in any of these key nutrients, it can significantly affect the thyroid function and could be slowing you and your metabolism right down.

Blood sugar balance is crucial to supporting optimum thyroid function. Many people with suboptimal thyroid function often feel quite unwell first thing in the morning, when our blood sugar levels are at their lowest. A protein-rich breakfast is advisable, and intermittent fasting, such as the 16:8 diet (where you eat within an 8-hour window and fast for the remaining time) can often prove unsuitable for people with an underactive thyroid. See page 113 for detailed advice on blood sugar management.

Protein

As we saw in Step 3, protein is the building block of life. Every cell, muscle, organ and gland in the body is made of protein – including the thyroid. Getting enough protein helps keep your thyroid strong and functioning properly.

Beyond overall thyroid health, there's another key reason to focus on protein: it contains the amino acid tyrosine, which combines with iodine to produce thyroid hormones. You can find out more about the different amino acids on pages 41–4.

Protein-rich foods are also often excellent sources of iron, another crucial nutrient for thyroid function (as you'll see below).

To best support your thyroid, aim to include protein in every meal and snack.

Food sources of protein
- **Animal sources:** meat, fish, eggs; concentrated forms of dairy, such as cottage cheese or authentic Greek yogurt (e.g. 9g/¼oz of protein per 100g/3½oz)
- **Plant sources:** pulses, e.g. lentils, chickpeas/garbanzo beans, or beans; soya, quinoa, nuts and seeds

See pages 46–7 for a table listing the protein content of foods per 100g and advice on portions.

Iodine

Iodine is a trace mineral which is required in only small amounts, but it is nevertheless essential for a healthy thyroid and to prevent the risk of goitre, which is a swollen thyroid gland. It also plays a key role in cognitive function. Historically, certain countries have had a high prevalence of goitre due to the lack of iodine in the soil, but the introduction of iodized salt in modern times has largely addressed this issue.

It's important to get the balance of iodine right, because too much can be as problematic for the thyroid as too little. Excessive iodine levels can actually inhibit the production of thyroid hormones and may also cause unpleasant symptoms, such as mouth sores, diarrhoea and vomiting.

The sensible approach for thyroid support would be to simply ensure that you're including iodine-rich foods in your diet on a regular basis. Any significant imbalances should be dealt with by your doctor.

Food sources of iodine

- Sea vegetables, e.g. kelp, nori or samphire
- Fish and seafood
- Dairy products (due to iodine-supplemented feed in cattle)
- Eggs

Iodine supplements

Due to the delicate balance required for iodine, it's essential to be very careful about supplementing it without the specific support of a health professional. It's not unusual for iodine to feature in very small quantities in a multivitamin and mineral supplement, but it's important not to supplement iodine in isolation without medical advice.

Iron

Iron deficiency is a key player in hypothyroidism, because of its role in the production of thyroxine (T4) and the conversion of T4 to T3. Low levels of iron could also impact thyroid-stimulating hormone (TSH) levels and may even impair the absorption of iodine.

This is an important nutrient to keep under review, because it's not unusual for perimenopausal women to be low in iron, due to heavy periods or flooding, which are a common issue during the hormonal fluctuations of the premenopausal stage.

Iron deficiency can cause fatigue in its own right, due to the role it plays in the production and delivery of energy to our body cells. A blood test from your doctor will help establish the status of iron in your blood. Supplements should be taken four hours away from any thyroid medication, because they could decrease absorption. For more information on factors that support or enhance the absorption of iron, as well as detailed advice on supplements and understanding test results, see page 147.

Food sources of iron

Top sources of iron include lean red meat (such as beef, lamb and venison), eggs and dark green leafy vegetables. See pages 155–7 for a detailed table of animal and plant sources of iron and for specific advice on supplements, which should be treated with caution.

B vitamins

B vitamins are a family of nutrients which work together to support our health and wellbeing, and they're particularly important for cognitive function, mood, mental health and energy. As we have seen in Step 1, they're key players in the chain reaction that produces the energy storage molecules ATP.

Vitamins B2, B3 and B6 all play an active part in the production of the thyroid hormone T4, so a B vitamin deficiency could be playing a part in your symptoms.

Food sources of B vitamins

These three B vitamins are found in most foods in small quantities, but here are some of the concentrated sources:

- **B2:** sunflower seeds, mushrooms, organ meat, fish, pulses and walnuts
- **B3:** wheat bran, white meat, brewer's yeast, broccoli
- **B6:** meat, eggs, dairy products, brewer's yeast, sunflower seeds

B vitamin supplements

These are best taken as part of a B vitamin complex, which contains the full range, due to the synergistic action of the B vitamin family. For more specific information and advice on B vitamins, see page 167.

Selenium

Selenium is an antioxidant mineral which plays a key role in supporting the immune function and protecting against the formation of the free radicals that often play a role in chronic health conditions. It works closely with vitamin E to support antibody production and to maintain a healthy heart and liver.

Selenium also plays an important role in thyroid metabolism, because it's required for the conversion from T4 to T3; it may also help to reduce thyroid antibody levels in cases of the autoimmune condition Hashimoto's thyroiditis.

As well as contributing to impaired thyroid function, a deficiency in selenium may lead to muscle weakness, fatigue and poor immune function.

Food sources of selenium

The most concentrated natural source of selenium is a Brazil nut. But it's important to apply moderation here: one Brazil nut contains roughly 140mcg of selenium, and the maximum daily recommended amount is 200mcg. Excessive levels of selenium may lead to toxicity. Brazil nuts may also contain the heavy metals barium and radium, due to the extremely deep roots of their trees, which is another good reason to only eat them in moderation, with no more than 1–2 per day to stay on the safe side.

Other food sources of selenium include meat, poultry, seafood, fish and some seeds.

Selenium supplements

Supplementation should be treated with caution, for the reasons set out above. Selenium usually features in a small dose in a multivitamin and mineral supplement, which is probably the most appropriate way to take it, because it works in synergy with other nutrients. It's not advisable to take selenium as a concentrated individual supplement without the advice of a health professional.

Zinc

Zinc is a powerful antioxidant that plays a key role in a whole range of bodily systems, including our reproductive organs, skin, liver function and immune system. It's crucial for the cascade of thyroid hormones, because it's required for the conversion of T4 to T3, which is the active thyroid hormone. We also need it for the absorption of vitamin E.

A deficiency in zinc can increase your susceptibility to infection, affect wound healing and lead to poor sense of taste or smell, hair loss and skin issues. It's also a common cause of white marks on fingernails.

Food sources of zinc

Zinc is found in most food in small quantities. These are some of the more concentrated sources: lamb, fish, oysters, walnuts, almonds, sardines, legumes.

Zinc supplements

It's important to avoid taking more than 25mg of zinc per day in supplement form without the advice of a health professional. Supplements are powerful things, and more is not necessarily better! In fact, doses of over 100mg daily of zinc can actually depress the immune function. It's also important to take zinc supplements at least two hours away from iron tablets, as they can interfere with each other's activity in the body.

Vitamin E

Vitamin E is a fat-soluble vitamin, which means that the body can store it for use when we need it. It's made up of eight different antioxidant compounds called tocopherols, which work in synergy. Vitamin E plays a key role in supporting our immune function and neutralizing the free radicals that increase the risk of conditions such as cancer or cardiovascular disease. We also need it for healthy, vibrant skin, which is why it's commonly known as the "anti-ageing" vitamin.

In thyroid terms, it's another nutrient required for the cascade that produces thyroid hormones.

Low levels of vitamin E may affect skin health and immune function, and impair the action of red blood cells.

Food sources of vitamin E

Vitamin E is found in small amounts in a broad range of foods and women need a minimum of 3mg per day from food sources. These are some concentrated sources of vitamin E: sunflower seeds, avocado, dark green leafy vegetables, legumes, peanuts, wheatgerm.

Vitamin E supplements

If you're choosing a vitamin E supplement, check the label for "mixed tocopherols". This means it contains the full range of vitamin E types, just as they occur in nature. These are likely to be more effective than supplements that only list alpha-tocopherol, which is just one type of vitamin E.

Excessive levels of vitamin E supplements may lead to toxicity, so it's important to respect the recommended dosage on the label. As with all supplements, you should consult your doctor before starting them if you're taking any medication or have any medical conditions, to avoid any potential harmful interactions.

Vitamin A

This is another group of fat-soluble nutrients. They consist of retinoids, which are found in animal sources – retinol is an example of this – and carotenoids, which are antioxidant plant compounds, such as beta-carotene. The body converts carotenoids into vitamin A in the liver.

We need vitamin A to support our immune function and to protect against infection. It's also important for healthy cell membranes, skin, hair and eye health.

A deficiency can lead to dry skin or acne, impaired night vision, mouth ulcers, fatigue and frequent colds and infections.

Retinol is required for the uptake of iodine in the body. We also need vitamin A for the manufacture of thyroid hormones and the optimal function of T3.

Food sources of vitamin A
- **Retinol:** chicken liver or calf liver, shellfish, egg yolk
- **Beta-carotene:** carrots, sweet potato, butternut squash, dark green leafy vegetables

Vitamin A supplements
Foods or supplements that are high in vitamin A are not recommended during pregnancy, although this is unlikely to be an issue if you are menopausal. Post-menopause, it's not advisable to be taking more than 1.5mg or 1500mcg (or μg) of vitamin A in supplement form per day. Always check with your doctor if you have any concerns.

Vitamin D
It's worth ensuring that your vitamin D levels are optimal, because of the very important role this vitamin plays in modulating and supporting the immune system, as well as its role in bone health.

Some studies have shown that a high proportion of people with the autoimmune condition Hashimoto's thyroiditis (a common cause of an underactive thyroid) have vitamin D deficiency. Optimal vitamin D levels may help to regulate levels of thyroid antibodies, if these are a concern.

While there is still a gap in knowledge as to the exact role and influence of vitamin D on thyroid health, the connection seems clear, so it's only logical to check that you don't have a vitamin D deficiency by asking your doctor for a blood test. Any imbalance can be easily remedied by vitamin D supplementation and may contribute positively to your thyroid health.

To understand more about the benefits of vitamin D, how we produce it in the body, food sources and supplements, see page 181.

Foods to limit for optimal thyroid health

Certain foods contain goitrogens, which are naturally occurring compounds that can interfere with the production of thyroid hormone, by blocking the uptake of iodine. This won't impact a healthy thyroid function, however if you have sub-clinical thyroid function, it is an area to bear in mind. You don't have to eliminate these foods altogether, but it would be wise to avoid large portions of goitrogenic foods on a daily basis.

Examples of foods that are high in goitrogens include soya beans and associated products such as tofu, tempeh or soya milk products, raw spinach and raw cruciferous vegetables, such as broccoli, kale or cabbage. Lightly cooked spinach or cruciferous vegetables should not be problematic, because the cooking process reduces the impact of the goitrogens in these foods.

If your underactive thyroid has been triggered by an autoimmune condition, such as Hashimoto's thyroiditis, you may find it helpful to eliminate gluten from your diet for six months and observe the potential impact. Some studies suggest that this can reduce the inflammatory load triggering the thyroid antibodies and may help to reduce TSH levels. A gluten-free diet may also support the effective absorption of vitamin D and selenium, which are both essential for thyroid function.

Lifestyle to support optimal thyroid health

Chronic stress is a common cause of thyroid dysfunction. Our adrenal glands, which produce our stress hormones and regulate our stress response, work closely with the hypothalamus and the pituitary gland in an alliance known as the HPA (hypothalamic–pituitary–adrenal) axis. Overworked adrenal glands will put pressure on this relationship and this can interfere with the thyroid–pituitary axis, affecting the production of TSH.

Stress may also impair the conversion process of T4 to the active thyroid hormone T3, diverting it to become reverse T3 instead, which is the inactive form of the hormone.

Cellular sensitivity to thyroid hormones can also be affected by high levels of stress hormones, which can reduce the ability of the hormone to enter the cell and do its work.

In short, if you're struggling with high levels of stress, this may be having a direct impact on the thyroid function.

How stressed are you? There are probably some quick fixes you can apply straightaway to help manage your adrenal load. Consider simple strategies, such as reviewing your schedule, so that you're not overloading yourself; daring to say "no", so that you don't take on too much in the way of work or caring responsibilities; and blocking out "me-time", so that you have a chance to take a breath.

Have a look at page 241 where I explore stress in more detail and explain the different ways that you can support the adrenal glands and regulate the body's response to stress, which may help to remove the pressure from your thyroid.

EXAMPLES OF THYROID-FRIENDLY FOODS TO PRIORITIZE IN YOUR DIET

Animal proteins	Vegetables	Nuts & seeds	Pulses	Grains
Lean red meat, e.g. grass-fed beef, venison, lamb; oily fish, e.g. sardines, salmon, mackerel; white fish; eggs	Dark green leafy veg, e.g. kale, spinach, chard, broccoli, rocket/arugula, watercress; butternut squash, orange or red peppers, courgette/zucchini, artichoke, mushrooms, tomatoes, carrots	Walnuts, almonds, Brazil nut (maximum 1–2 daily), ground flaxseed, pumpkin seeds, sunflower seeds, chia seeds, hemp	Lentils, chickpeas/garbanzo beans, butter/lima beans, broad/fava beans, haricot/navy beans, kidney beans, cannellini beans, split peas	Brown rice, quinoa, buckwheat, corn

EXAMPLES OF THYROID-FRIENDLY MEALS

Breakfast	Lunch	Dinner	Snacks
2 eggs with ½ avocado and lightly cooked spinach	Gluten-free sourdough or wrap with houmous, falafel, red onion and green salad	Quinoa with cubes of roasted butternut squash, red onion, red pepper and courgettes/zucchini	1 Brazil nut with an apple
Chia seed pudding or 160g authentic natural Greek yogurt (9g protein per 100g), with 35g mixed pumpkin and sunflower seeds, and 100g blueberries or chopped apple	Salad with a grilled chicken breast or 160g pulses with rocket/arugula, watercress, tomatoes and grated carrot, sprinkled with pumpkin seeds	Lamb chops with broccoli, carrots and roasted cherry tomatoes	2 rough oatcakes with almond butter or mackerel pâté

CASE STUDY: Overcoming an underactive thyroid – Tracy's story

Tracy, 47, came to my clinic during perimenopause. HRT had eased her hot flushes and low mood, but she was still struggling with extreme fatigue and weight gain she couldn't shift. Once full of energy, she now lacked the stamina for even a short walk and felt frustrated and written off as "just another menopausal woman".

During her consultation, it became clear that her symptoms – particularly the fatigue and weight gain – aligned with an underactive thyroid. I wrote to her doctor requesting a blood test, and the results confirmed the diagnosis.

With two months of thyroid medication, along with the dietary changes I recommended, Tracy's energy returned, she was back to hiking, and her weight began to drop. She finally felt like herself again.

Easy ways to support your thyroid function

- Ensure that you have at least one complete protein in your diet every day. See page 45 for advice on complete proteins.
- Optimize your iron absorption by drinking tea or coffee two hours away from a meal.
- Boost your dietary iodine by treating yourself to sea vegetables once a week.
- Steer clear of large portions of soya, if you suspect you have an underactive thyroid.
- Eat a rainbow of different-coloured vegetables across the week to access the different antioxidants that support your thyroid gland.
- Consider a gluten-free diet for a six-month period.
- Modulate your stress levels by managing your schedule more carefully.

Energy Action Plan – my next steps

What three things are you going to do to support your thyroid function, if you think it's a potential concern for you? They might involve speaking to your doctor to arrange a test; perhaps there are certain foods you need to focus on or avoid; and is there a lifestyle change that you think would be beneficial?

Make a note of whatever stood out to you in this section and create a commitment to tackling the issue.

Focus on these three questions to create your SMART objectives:

1. What will I do?
2. How will I do it?
3. When will I do it by?

YOUR GUIDE TO IRON

Quiz 3 (see page 107) was all about symptoms frequently associated with low levels of iron.

Iron is an important mineral which is a key player in the energy production process, because of its role in the production of haemoglobin and myoglobin. Haemoglobin is the protein in our red blood cells that carries oxygen around the body to fuel the activity of our cells, tissues, muscles and brain. Myoglobin is a form of haemoglobin required for efficient functioning of our muscles.

As we have seen in Step 1, it's essential for oxygen to reach every body cell in order to create the ATP energy storage units that we need for physical and mental strength, speed and stamina.

When we eat foods that are rich in iron, they are mostly absorbed in the small intestine. Once the iron is taken into the bloodstream, it's bound to a carrier protein called transferrin and transported to the bone marrow to produce red blood cells. It takes about a week for a red blood cell to fully mature and be released to carry out its principal role of delivering oxygen around the body. The average lifespan of a red blood cell is four months, which is why there is a continual renewal process.

Many people automatically assume that low energy is due to iron deficiency anaemia and decide to take iron tablets. In fact, there are multiple reasons why you might experience fatigue, and the process of iron metabolism is complex, so it's important to ensure that you have a diagnosis before making a unilateral decision to take supplements.

The human body can't excrete iron, in the way that it does with excess levels of some other nutrients. If there's too much iron in the body, it may build up in your tissues, potentially damaging the digestive tract and causing symptoms of nausea, vomiting, diarrhoea and pain.

How does iron deficiency affect my energy levels?

Low levels of iron can lead to a condition known as iron deficiency anaemia, which will affect red blood cell production and may reduce levels of haemoglobin in the blood. This in turn will reduce the amount of oxygen transported to your body cells, so that they can't perform their normal functions. Anaemia can affect you in a variety of different ways, including muscular weakness, impaired cell repair and regeneration, and a lack of oxygen reaching the brain can cause dizziness and affect cognitive function. Adequate iron levels are also essential for effective mitochondrial function, supporting the action of the electron transport phase of energy production (see page 290) and the generation of ATP energy molecules.

Typical signs of iron deficiency anaemia

- Weakness
- Lack of stamina
- Fatigue
- Breathlessness
- Dizziness
- Pale skin
- Headaches
- Palpitations
- Sore tongue
- Brittle or thinning hair
- Loss of appetite

Why might the menopause affect my iron levels?

The most common cause of iron deficiency anaemia is blood loss. The hormonal fluctuations of the perimenopause can cause many women to experience heavier periods or even flooding. It's also not unusual for periods to last much longer, so the blood loss can be more extensive.

A more roundabout potential link is a reduced ability to absorb iron. Some women experience issues with acid reflux in midlife and may be using over-the-counter antacids on a regular basis or be taking prescribed medication, such as omeprazole, to reduce acid levels in the stomach. Low levels of stomach acid impair iron absorption, so this could be a contributory factor in your fatigue.

Potential causes of iron deficiency anaemia

- Blood loss
- A vegan or largely plant-based diet
- Prolonged use of antacids
- Drinking too much tea or coffee
- Low levels of vitamins B6 or B12, which can affect iron absorption
- High levels of phytates (wheat, bran or oats) or oxalates (spinach or rhubarb) in the diet, which may block iron absorption

UNDERSTANDING YOUR TEST RESULTS

If you suspect you may be low in iron, it's very important to speak to your doctor about a blood test, rather than assuming this is the cause of your fatigue and taking iron tablets. As we have seen above, this may be counterproductive if you're not actually low in iron.

It's not always easy to understand blood test results and there are a few different factors to take into account when assessing iron levels, so it's very important to get all the information.

The most likely areas that your doctor will investigate are haemoglobin (as part of a full blood count, which also includes testing levels of red blood cells, white blood cells and platelets), serum ferritin, total iron and transferrin saturation. It's the overall picture from these results that will determine the appropriate course of action.

As with other blood tests, the reference range for "normal", which is statistically based on a group of healthy people, tends to be very broad. But what is normal for other people may not be normal for you, if you find yourself at the lower end of the scale. It's also important to recognize that there can be quite a grey area between normal and optimal. If you're feeling very tired, you may find that your symptoms improve significantly by achieving optimal levels of iron in your system.

You can see below what the different scales are and where your test results might sit in relation to an optimal level.

Haemoglobin

Testing haemoglobin levels is just one part of the picture. Low levels of haemoglobin alone would not be sufficient to warrant iron tablets, without testing ferritin and total iron levels. For example, it's possible to have high ferritin and low haemoglobin if something is affecting the production of haemoglobin in the bone marrow (an example of this could be a medical treatment, such as chemotherapy). If this were the case, supplementing iron tablets would absolutely not be recommended, because this is not iron deficiency anaemia. Taking iron tablets unnecessarily could lead to excessive stores of iron building up in the tissues.

Blood levels of haemoglobin are usually reported as grams per litre (g/L) or grams per decilitre (g/dL), depending on the laboratory used by your doctor.

For women, the optimal range of haemoglobin is: 135–155g/L or 13.5–15.5g/dL

While slightly higher levels can be safe, levels above 155 g/L may indicate dehydration or underlying conditions and should be checked by a doctor.

Ferritin

Ferritin is a protein that stores iron in your body and releases it when needed to help produce red blood cells in the bone marrow. A serum ferritin test measures how much iron is stored in your tissues.

Ferritin would usually be reported in your results as either nanograms per millilitre (ng/mL) or micrograms per litre (mcg/L or µg/L).

For women, the optimal range of ferritin is: 70–90ng/mL or 70–90mcg/L (70–90µg/L).

While slightly higher levels can be safe, levels consistently above 150 µg/L may indicate iron overload and should be assessed by a doctor.

Total or serum iron

This reflects the total concentration of iron in the body. It's usually measured as micromoles per litre (µmol/L) or micrograms per decilitre (µg/dL).

For women, the optimal range is 20–30µmol/L or 111–170ug/dL

Higher serum iron levels may indicate iron overload or liver issues and should be evaluated by a doctor to avoid potential long-term tissue damage.

Transferrin saturation

Transferrin is a protein that regulates the amount of iron in the blood and moves it around the body. The saturation level reflects the amount of iron that is bound to transferrin. It's usually expressed as a percentage, or sometimes as a decimal of a percentage.

For women, the optimal range is 35% or 0.35.

Transferrin saturation above 45–50% is generally considered too high and warrants further investigation to prevent potential damage from excess iron, which can affect organs like the liver and heart.

The secret of red blood

The red colour in red blood cells is created when iron reacts to oxygen in the cell, during the energy production process.

HOW TO ACHIEVE OPTIMAL LEVELS OF IRON

Iron features in two forms in our diet: haem iron, which is found in animal sources, and non-haem iron, which is found in plant sources. Haem iron is more effectively absorbed by the body than non-haem iron, which can make vegetarians or vegans more susceptible to iron deficiency anaemia.

Compared with haem iron, non-haem iron from food sources tends to be more affected by other factors. For example, vitamin C can boost the absorption of non-haem iron by up to 30 per cent, while compounds found in coffee and tea can block its absorption. In contrast, haem iron doesn't require additional help from other nutrients and isn't significantly affected by inhibitors.

However, calcium supplements may interfere with the absorption of both haem and non-haem dietary iron, so it's best to take these two hours away from mealtimes.

Dietary requirements will vary, depending on whether you're still having regular periods or not. The recommended daily amount of dietary iron for menstruating women is 14.8mg; for non-menstruating women it is 8.7mg.

Lean red meat is a particularly good source of iron, as is offal, such as chicken or calf livers, although I would be wary of processed forms, such as liver pâté. Oily fish, such as sardines or tuna, are a decent source. White meat and white fish do contain iron, but significantly less, although of course they have other health benefits. While you may not want to be eating large amounts of red meat for wider health reasons, if your iron levels are low, it might be sensible to include it in your diet a couple of times per week, along with oily fish.

As you can see from the table opposite, there is a wide range of plant-based sources of iron per 100g serving. However, while certain foods may seem promising, 100g/3½oz represents an unusually large portion in some cases, which means you might not be getting as much iron as you think in a single serving. Ensuring a variety of iron-rich foods throughout the day is the most effective way to meet your daily recommended intake.

EVERYDAY FOODS THAT ARE GOOD SOURCES OF IRON

Haem iron content per 100g	Non-haem iron content per 100g
Meat	**Pulses**
Calf's liver 12.2mg	Lentils 2.4mg
Chicken liver 11.3mg	Chickpeas/garbanzo beans (canned) 1.5mg
Venison 5.1mg	Soya beans 3.0mg
Rump steak 3.6mg	Kidney beans (canned) 2.0mg
Beef mince 2.7mg	Butter/lima beans (canned) 1.5mg
Lamb chop 2.5mg	Baked beans (canned) 1.4mg
Pork chop 0.7mg	**Nuts**
Chicken breast 0.5mg	Almonds 3.0mg
Turkey breast 0.5mg	Hazelnuts 3.2mg
Fish	Walnuts 2.9mg
Sardines (canned) 2.7mg	**Seeds**
Mackerel (canned) 1.3mg	Pumpkin seeds 10mg
Tuna (canned) 1.5mg	Chia seeds 9.5mg
Salmon 0.5mg	Flaxseed 8.5mg
Sea bass 0.3mg	Sunflower seeds 6.4mg
Cod 0.2mg	**Soya**
Eggs & dairy	Tofu 3.5mg
Egg yolk (boiled) 6.2mg	Soya milk 0.43mg
Cheddar cheese 0.3mg	**Vegetables**
Yogurt 0.1mg	Parsley 7.7mg
Milk 0.02mg	Watercress 2.2mg
	Baby spinach 1.9mg
	Peas 1.8mg
	Kale 1.7mg
	Broccoli 0.8mg

EXAMPLES OF IRON-RICH MEALS

Breakfast	Lunch	Dinner	Snacks
2 poached eggs or scrambled tofu with wilted spinach	Wholemeal bread sandwich with falafel and houmous, or roast beef and salad	Lentil or lamb shepherd's pie with mixed green vegetables	15g almonds with a piece of fresh fruit
Natural yogurt or soya yogurt with fresh fruit and 2 table-spoons of pumpkin seeds	Watercress and kale salad, with sardines or crispy tofu	Venison sausages with sweet potato mash and peas	30g edamame beans

Iron supplements

Iron supplements should be treated with caution. While they may be easily available to buy over the counter, these are powerful products which contain a concentrated dose of iron. They should only be used if a blood test has identified your iron levels as low. The body has no mechanism for excreting excess iron. If you are taking iron supplements unnecessarily, any surplus iron will be stored in the tissues, which could generate unpleasant symptoms and may, over time, lead to a state of toxicity.

If your blood tests show sub-optimal iron levels, rather than an actual deficiency, your doctor may not prescribe iron tablets. If you decide to take a short-term dose of supplements, to optimize the levels, it's important to take another blood test after three months, to assess any changes in the results. This will inform the decision about further supplementation and ensure you are not taking them unnecessarily. A short-term course of iron tablets may significantly improve your energy levels, if you are running low. However, if you have any doubts or concerns, you should always seek advice from a medical professional.

Understanding the different iron tablets

There are a variety of iron tablets available. Inorganic forms of iron, such as ferrous sulphate, can be much harder for the body to absorb and can commonly cause digestive discomfort. Organic forms of iron are generally easier for the body to absorb; examples of these include ferrous fumarate, ferrous citrate or ferrous gluconate.

Sensitive individuals may find that most forms of iron supplements affect their digestion. If this is the case, it can sometimes be gentler on the stomach to take the tablet in the middle of the meal, rather than before or after. It's also possible to take a transdermal form of iron, via an oral spray that is absorbed through the skin of the cheek, rather than passing through the digestive system. This can help to reduce any unpleasant digestive symptoms.

Tea and coffee contain compounds that can affect the absorption of iron, so it's advisable to take iron tablets at least two hours away from these drinks. Iron tablets may interfere with thyroid medication, so it's best to leave a four-hour gap before taking them. Antacids should be taken two hours away from supplements, to maximize iron absorption.

Always respect the dosage on the label, because this will be carefully calculated in relation to the absorbability of the form of iron used. You should not exceed a daily dosage of 17mg of iron in supplement form without the supervision of a health professional.

CASE STUDY: The power of iron – Clare's story

Clare, 47, came to my clinic feeling constantly tired. Although she initially sought help for her IBS, it became clear that her fatigue was taking a serious toll. Juggling work, two children and caring responsibilities, she assumed her exhaustion was just part of life.

While addressing her digestive issues, I suspected her heavy periods and flooding might be causing iron deficiency anaemia. A referral to her doctor confirmed very low iron levels. Unfortunately, the prescribed iron tablets aggravated her IBS, so I recommended an oral spray that bypassed the gut. I also encouraged her to prioritize animal sources of iron, as they're more easily absorbed.

Once her iron levels began to normalize, Clare couldn't believe the difference – her energy returned, and she felt like a whole new woman!

Easy ways to optimize your iron levels

- Eat lean pasture-fed red meat twice a week, and try the occasional more unusual option, such as venison or calf's liver.
- Aim to consume a haem source of iron every day.
- Avoid drinking tea and coffee with meals or when you're taking iron tablets, to optimize absorption.
- Eat a couple of handfuls of dark green leafy vegetables every day.
- Enhance plant sources of iron by eating them with foods that are rich in vitamin C, such as red peppers, berries, green vegetables or citrus fruits.
- Avoid taking iron tablets and antacids within two hours of each other, to ensure you get the full benefit.

Energy Action Plan – my next steps

What three things are you going to do to support your iron levels, if you think it's a potential concern for you? They might involve speaking to your doctor to arrange a blood test; perhaps there are certain foods you need to focus on or avoid; and what could you do to optimize iron absorption?

Make a note of whatever stood out to you in this section and create a commitment to tackling the issue.

Focus on these three questions to create your SMART objectives:

1. What will I do?
2. How will I do it?
3. When will I do it by?

YOUR GUIDE TO VITAMIN B12

If you scored highly in Quiz 4 (see page 108), this may indicate an issue with your vitamin B12 levels. A deficiency is a very common cause of fatigue.

Vitamin B12 is a complex nutrient made up of biological compounds known as cobalamins. These cobalamins are part of the broader B vitamin family, which includes B1, B2, B3, B5, B6 and B9 (folate), all of which contribute to various essential functions in the body. We need B12 for the optimal digestion and absorption of food, and for energy metabolism. It also plays a part in cellular health and longevity.

How does vitamin B12 affect my energy levels?

Vitamin B12 is very important for our energy levels, because of the role it plays in the production of red blood cells and the transportation of oxygen to each cell in the body. It also supports the effective absorption of iron.

Effective mitochondrial function relies on optimal levels of vitamin B12 and a deficiency can impact the production of mitochondrial DNA and impair energy metabolism.

Vitamin B12 plays a key role in the health of our nervous system and it's essential for memory, learning and overall cognitive function. It influences our mood and mental health, and a deficiency can lead to anxiety or depression.

Low levels of vitamin B12 can impair the shape and size of red blood cells, affecting their ability to carry oxygen and this can lead to a form of anaemia which will leave you feeling extremely tired and low most of the time. This is why your doctor is likely to test blood levels if you complain of low energy and fatigue.

A vegan, plant-based or flexitarian diet may increase the risk of vitamin B12 deficiency, because it is only found in animal sources – meat, fish, eggs and dairy. Some forms of algae or seaweed contain vitamin B12, but it's unclear how easily absorbed this form would be and it's not currently considered a reliable source for dietary requirements. Certain fortified products include vitamin B12, but this may not be in sufficient amounts for optimal health and wellbeing.

Vegans and vegetarians should keep an eye on B12 blood levels and would probably benefit from supplementing.

Typical signs of vitamin B12 deficiency

- Exhaustion
- Poor memory
- Brain fog
- Low mood or depression
- Irritability
- Dizziness
- Headaches
- Sore tongue
- Shallow breathing
- Ringing in the ears
- Digestive problems

Why might the menopause affect my B12 levels?

The hormonal fluctuations around the perimenopause and menopause are unlikely to directly deplete vitamin B12. However, it's relatively common for women to experience digestive disturbances during this period, which could be a key contributory factor in depleting B12. For example, you may find that you're more prone to IBS symptoms such as bloating, loose stools or constipation. Hormonal changes may also affect the optimal balance of beneficial bacteria in the gut, which could generally impair nutrient absorption.

Problems of indigestion or acid reflux also often emerge around the menopause, which may lead to the use of antacid medication. This could directly affect the absorption of vitamin B12 and is a common cause of depletion.

A hidden deficiency?
The body can store vitamin B12 for 2–5 years, so it may take some time for a dietary deficiency to show.

Potential causes of vitamin B12 depletion

- A vegan or largely plant-based diet
- Malabsorption in the digestive tract due to an inflammatory bowel condition, such as Crohn's disease
- Stress
- Regular alcohol consumption
- Consistent use of antacid medication
- Pernicious anaemia, an autoimmune condition that affects the absorption of B12 in the stomach
- Low levels of vitamin B6, which can affect the absorption of B12
- Certain medication, such as metformin

UNDERSTANDING YOUR TEST RESULTS

If you explain your symptoms to your doctor, they will probably refer you for a total serum B12 test, which shows the total levels of B12 in the blood. B12 is likely to be measured in picomoles per litre (pmol/L), picograms per litre (pg/mL) or nanograms per millitre (ng/mL).

A deficiency would be considered as anything less than 118pmol/L, 180pg/mL or 180ng/mL in your test results and your doctor would prescribe corrective supplements.

However, these are very low levels of vitamin B12 indeed. If your test results are above these deficiency reference ranges, but not within an optimal range, a lack of vitamin B12 could still be at the root of your fatigue. It is likely that you would benefit from increasing dietary vitamin B12 and possibly using supplements as an extra support.

Optimal levels of serum vitamin B12 are:

700–1,000pmol/L, 948–1,355ng/L or 948–1,355pg/mL

HOW TO ACHIEVE OPTIMAL LEVELS OF VITAMIN B12

VITAMIN B12 CONTENT OF EVERYDAY FOODS PER 100G

Meat

Lamb's liver 83mcg

Chicken liver 45mcg

Beef 2.5mcg

Lamb 2.5mcg

Ham 1mcg

Pork 1mcg

Chicken 1mcg

Turkey 1mcg

Eggs

Chicken egg 2mcg

Fortified foods per serving

Yeast extract spread (per 8g) 1.5mcg

Fortified bran flakes (per 30g) 0.69mcg

Fortified corn flakes (per 30g) 0.57mcg

Fish

Sardines 9mcg

Mackerel 8.7mcg

Salmon 3mcg

Tuna 3mcg

Cod 2mcg

Haddock 2mcg

Dairy

Cheddar cheese 1.3mcg

Feta cheese 1.1mcg

Cow's milk 0.9mcg

Natural yogurt 0.3mcg

Brie 0.6mcg

Cottage cheese 0.3mcg

EXAMPLES OF VITAMIN-B12-RICH MEALS

Breakfast	Lunch	Dinner	Snacks
2 eggs on wholemeal toast	Wholemeal bread sandwich with roast beef and horseradish	Grilled sardines with roasted vegetables	Carrot sticks with mackerel pâté
Fortified bran flakes with cow's milk or a slice of wholemeal toast with marmite	Warm chicken liver salad	Feta cheese and vegetable omelette	1–2 rough oatcakes with smoked salmon

Vitamin B12 supplements

If a blood test reveals that your vitamin B12 levels are sufficiently low, your doctor may prescribe a B12 supplement for a period of time, before retesting to assess the situation.

If you have tested positive for the autoimmune condition pernicious anaemia, simply increasing dietary vitamin B12 will not be sufficient to correct the issue, because you will be unable to absorb it. Your doctor is likely to recommend regular B12 injections or a tablet that dissolves under the tongue and absorbs through the skin, to ensure the appropriate balance is maintained.

If your blood levels are deemed to be within the normal range, but don't fall within the optimal range (see above), you may benefit from taking supplements for a short period of time.

It's important not to take high individual doses of vitamin B12 without the advice a trained health professional. This could disrupt the optimal balance of B vitamins in the body, which may do more harm than good.

What to look for in a B vitamin supplement

It's advisable to choose a B vitamin complex supplement that contains a methylated form of vitamin B12 (e.g. methylcobalamin), because this tends to be more easily absorbed and is therefore more effective.

Certain supplements provide B12 in the form of cyanocobalamin, which is a cheaper form of the nutrient that may not be absorbed by the body as easily, so may not be as supportive of your energy levels.

Once your energy levels improve, the supplement may no longer be required and you can continue to support optimal B12 levels by following a balanced diet. After about six months, it's advisable to request a further blood test, to assess your B12 status and ensure levels are not excessive.

About the B vitamin family

Although this section focuses on vitamin B12, it's helpful to understand the role of the broader B vitamin family. These are a group of distinct nutrients, each with a specific role in supporting the body and categorized by a numbering system from 1 to 12. Not all numbers are used, as some nutrients were later discovered not to be vitamins.

These vitamins work together to support overall health and wellbeing in various ways, and they are especially important for physical and mental energy. A deficiency in one B vitamin can often indicate a deficiency in another, which is why using a B vitamin complex, containing the appropriate doses of all the different B vitamins rather than individual doses, is generally recommended to ensure balance and synergy.

As we discovered in Step 1, B vitamins play a crucial role in the chain reaction of energy production. B1 (thiamine), B2 (riboflavin), B3 (niacin) and B5 (pantothenic acid) are key players in ATP production. Meanwhile, B12, B9 (folate) and B6 contribute to red blood cell production, oxygen transportion to cells and supporting the effective absorption of iron. Vitamin B6 also enhances the absorption of B12.

Certain B vitamins are also essential for mood, mental clarity and cognitive function. For example, B1 (thiamine) supports memory and learning capacity; B3 (niacin) is important for brain function and memory; B5 helps reduce stress levels by supporting adrenal function; B6 acts as a natural antidepressant by supporting serotonin production; and B9 (folate) plays a critical role in neurological development and overall brain health.

It's clear how vital all B vitamins are in maintaining both physical and mental health and energy, which is why a combination supplement in the form of a B vitamin complex often provides the most effective support.

B vitamin	Function	Food sources
B1 (Thiamine)	Supports energy metabolism and nerve function	Whole grains, legumes, nuts, pork
B2 (Riboflavin)	Aids in energy production and skin health	Dairy, eggs, green leafy vegetables
B3 (Niacin)	Important for brain function and cardiovascular health	Meat, poultry, fish, nuts
B5 (Pantothenic Acid)	Supports hormone synthesis and stress management	Avocado, mushrooms, whole grains
B6 (Pyridoxine)	Vital for red blood cell production, protein metabolism and mood regulation	Poultry, fish, potatoes, bananas
B7 (Biotin)	Essential for skin, hair health and metabolism	Eggs, nuts, seeds, spinach
B9 (Folate)	Important for DNA synthesis, red blood cell production and neurological health	Leafy greens, legumes, fortified cereals

CASE STUDY: Beating burnout with vitamin B12 – Angela's story

Angela, 50, came to see me feeling overwhelmed, anxious, jittery and completely drained. With so much stress in her life, it seemed likely her B vitamin levels had been depleted, which is very common for women in midlife, in my experience. After a blood test revealed her B12 levels were suboptimal – not low enough for injections, but insufficient to support sustained energy – I worked with her to increase her intake of B vitamins through diet and adjusted her cooking methods to prevent nutrient loss, as B vitamins are water-soluble and easily depleted by boiling or long cooking times. In addition, I recommended a three-month course of a high-dose B vitamin complex, with a follow-up test planned. Within weeks, Angela reported feeling much more resilient, and over several months, we continued working together to get her fully back on track.

Easy ways to optimize your vitamin B12 levels

- Aim to eat foods from an animal source several times a week.
- Consider supplementing with a B vitamin complex if you're a vegan or follow a largely plant-based diet.
- Ensure that you're using the most absorbable form of vitamin B12 supplement.
- Reduce your alcohol consumption.
- Opt for good-quality, unprocessed fortified foods.

Energy Action Plan – my next steps

What three things can you do to support your vitamin B12 levels, if you think this is a potential concern for you? Perhaps you need to consult your doctor for a blood test, if you suspect that you may be deficient. You may benefit from addressing the balance of your diet to include more foods from animal sources. Could it be time to think about supplements?

Make a note of whatever stood out to you in this section and create a commitment to tackling the issue.

Focus on these three questions to create your SMART objectives:

1. What will I do?
2. How will I do it?
3. When will I do it by?

YOUR GUIDE TO MAGNESIUM

If you scored highly in Quiz 5 (see page 109), then it's time to learn more about magnesium, because it could be the culprit in your fatigue.

Magnesium is a very busy mineral which is responsible for over 300 different biochemical reactions in the body and associated with hundreds more. This multi-tasking role makes it a key player in our health and wellbeing, because it's crucial for the effective functioning of so many important bodily systems.

And yet, when people are considering a potential deficiency, magnesium is often overlooked in favour of other minerals, such as iron or calcium. This is partly because the symptoms of magnesium deficiency can be quite insidious, and may have started early in life, precisely when we should be building up reserves to support a strong skeleton. A recent study suggested that teenage girls were only consuming 53 per cent of the magnesium they needed in their diet.

Tired, aching muscles can be associated with magnesium deficiency. We also need it for peristalsis, which is the contraction of the bowel muscle as it pushes a stool through our digestive tract. Low levels could lead to constipation, bloating and irregular bowel movements.

Magnesium can also help to play a role in managing chronic pain and relieving or reducing the severity of headaches or migraines. We need magnesium to support the absorption of calcium and to build strong bones. It's also important for cardiovascular function and supporting a healthy blood pressure.

If you're low in magnesium, you're likely to feel absolutely worn out, quite jittery or anxious, and it may feel as if you're just clinging on by your fingertips and operating on sheer willpower. This is because magnesium is absolutely vital for the energy production process in the body and the effective functioning of the nervous system.

How does magnesium support my energy levels?

Energy production in the body involves a complex sequence of chain reactions. Magnesium activates the enzymes that set off this whole process, which means that without it, you won't even get off the starting blocks. It also plays a key role in the production of ATP energy molecules in the citric acid cycle (see page 289). Without sufficient magnesium, the efficiency of mitochondrial energy production decreases, depleting energy levels and leading to fatigue.

Magnesium is important for nerve and muscle impulses, so a deficiency can cause anxiety, irritability and nervousness. It's nature's calmer, supporting our nervous system and regulating the body's response to stress, so we feel better equipped to cope with the challenges of daily life.

Optimum levels of magnesium can help to reduce the risk of low mood, depression, dizziness and pre-menstrual syndrome (PMS).

Typical signs of magnesium deficiency

- Persistent low energy
- Fatigue
- Muscle cramps, twitches or spasms
- Aching muscles or joints
- Palpitations
- Anxiety, irritability or nervousness
- Constipation
- Insomnia
- Headaches or migraines

Why might the menopause affect my magnesium levels?

There isn't a direct link between menopause and magnesium depletion, but the context of midlife can contribute to factors that may affect magnesium levels. For instance, the complex challenges that often accompany this phase – such as increased stress (see page 241) – can lead to higher magnesium depletion.

Additionally, many women begin taking calcium supplements to support bone health. However, high doses of calcium can interfere with magnesium absorption.

It's also common to experience acid reflux during menopause. Antacid tablets or proton pump inhibitor medications may further reduce magnesium absorption, so it may be advisable to take them two hours away from magnesium supplements.

Potential causes of magnesium depletion

- Chronic stress
- High-dose calcium supplements, which can decrease magnesium absorption
- Dietary deficiency
- Excessive alcohol consumption
- Digestive problems affecting nutrient absorption
- Certain medication, such as antibiotics, diuretics, antacids or steroids, which can increase the need for magnesium
- Too many fizzy drinks containing phosphoric acid, which can impair absorption

Testing for magnesium

A magnesium blood test isn't on the usual roster of tests that you'd get from your doctor and doesn't feature within the standard full blood count test. It's actually pretty difficult to test effectively for magnesium, because about 99 per cent of it is held in soft tissue or bone, with only about 1 per cent found in the blood. It's so important to our health and wellbeing that the body holds onto it strenuously, so a blood test may not be terribly revealing.

Magnesium depletion can gradually develop and is often difficult to pinpoint due to its involvement in numerous bodily systems. Symptoms can be varied, making it a challenge to identify low magnesium levels until a clearer pattern emerges.

HOW TO ACHIEVE OPTIMAL LEVELS OF MAGNESIUM

We require a minimum of 300mg of magnesium from food daily, which can generally be achieved through a wholefoods diet. Magnesium is present in a variety of wholefoods, with dark green leafy vegetables being one of the top sources. These are also rich in menopause-friendly nutrients, such as B vitamins, iron, calcium, vitamin C and vitamin K, making them an excellent choice. Wholegrain foods such as brown rice, rye and quinoa are also great sources, along with nuts and seeds, meat, fish and tofu.

MAGNESIUM CONTENT OF EVERYDAY VEGETABLES PER 100G		
Food	**Raw**	**Cooked**
Swiss chard	81mg	81mg
Baby spinach	80mg	54mg
Okra	57mg	40mg
Kale	47mg	23mg
Rocket/arugula	47mg	Not generally cooked
Watercress	38mg	Not generally cooked
Peas	33mg	24mg
Green beans	25mg	20mg
Broccoli	21mg	19mg
Courgette/zucchini	17mg	13mg
Green cabbage	13mg	14mg

MAGNESIUM CONTENT OF EVERYDAY WHOLEGRAINS PER 100G

Wholemeal bread 66mg	Brown rice 48mg
Quinoa 64mg	Porridge/oatmeal 28mg
Rye bread 40mg	Wholewheat pasta 21mg

MAGNESIUM CONTENT OF EVERYDAY PROTEIN SOURCES PER 100G

Animal protein sources	Plant protein sources
Fish	**Soya**
Sardines 40mg	Tofu 67mg
Tuna 35mg	Soya bean 63mg
Salmon 30mg	**Pulses**
Cod 30mg	Chickpeas/garbanzo beans 37mg
Plaice 22mg	Baked beans 30mg
Meat	Butter/lima beans 27mg
Chicken breast 36mg	Lentils 26mg
Turkey breast 30mg	**Nuts & seeds**
Beef 22mg	Brazil nuts 410mg
Lamb 21mg	Almonds 270mg
Dairy & eggs	Cashews 250mg
Cheddar 29mg	Walnuts 160mg
Natural yogurt 16mg	Hazelnuts 150mg
Milk 11mg	Sunflower seeds 390mg
Egg 14mg	Chia seeds 335mg
	Ground flaxseed 310mg
	Pumpkin seeds 270mg

EXAMPLES OF MAGNESIUM-RICH MEALS

Breakfast	Lunch	Dinner	Snacks
Natural yogurt with fresh fruit and 1 tablespoon each sunflower seeds and ground flaxseed	Wholemeal bread sandwich with salmon and watercress	Quinoa with roasted vegetables	1–2 oatcakes with houmous
Chia seed pudding with soya milk and blueberries	Baby spinach salad with sardines or edamame beans	Tofu or chicken stir-fry with Swiss chard, cashew nuts and courgette/zucchini	15g almonds with an apple

Magnesium supplements

If you think that magnesium supplements might be suitable for you, there are a few things to consider. Firstly, you must check with your doctor if you're taking any medication, or have any medical conditions, before you start taking oral magnesium. Excessive levels of magnesium may lower blood pressure and lead to light headedness; loose stools or diarrhoea are another common side effect of too much magnesium.

Magnesium comes in different forms of supplements; some of the most common are oxides, sulphates, chlorides, citrates, malates or glycinates. It's important to identify the form that suits you best, because some are more easily absorbed than others.

Our ability to absorb magnesium is dependent on the strength of the bond within the magnesium compound. Magnesium oxide, for example, contains the highest level of magnesium, which might seem very positive. However, it also has the strongest bond which makes it very difficult to break down, so that you'd actually be getting very little of the potential benefit from a magnesium oxide tablet.

The more effective forms tend to be citrates, malates or glycinates. These contain less elemental magnesium than an oxide form, but are much more easily absorbed by the gut, so would be a more beneficial option in oral supplement form. Some sensitive individuals may find magnesium citrate causes loose stools, although that could also be a helpful option for anyone who is prone to a sluggish bowel or constipation.

It's also possible to benefit from transdermal magnesium, commonly found in sulphates (e.g. Epsom salts) or chlorides, as bath salts. There are also a number of excellent magnesium skin sprays and lotions available, for topical use. Transdermal magnesium will be absorbed through the skin rather than the gut, so this can be an effective way of avoiding any digestive issues or medication interactions you might experience with an oral supplement.

To enjoy a magnesium sulphate or chloride bath, add 2–3 handfuls of salts to a bath or footbath and soak for at least 20 minutes. This is an excellent way to top up your magnesium levels, ease any muscle tension and set you up for a great night's sleep.

Oral magnesium supplements should not exceed 400mg daily without the advice of a health professional. Transdermal magnesium via a spray, lotion or bath salts may be taken in addition to this.

CASE STUDY: Restoring sleep & energy – Emma's story

Emma, 51, came to my clinic feeling constantly fatigued, with muscle cramps, trouble sleeping and persistent stress. She had tried everything, but nothing seemed to help. I suspected magnesium deficiency, which can lead to all these symptoms. I recommended magnesium-rich foods and suggested she take a magnesium supplement in the evenings to help with sleep and muscle relaxation. I also advised regular Epsom salts baths. Within just a few weeks of adding magnesium to her diet and supplementing at night, Emma felt a noticeable improvement. Her energy levels rose, her muscle cramps disappeared, and she was sleeping soundly. She also felt less stressed and better equipped to cope with her daily challenges. Magnesium really is a brilliant all-rounder!

Easy ways to optimize your magnesium levels

- Eat two handfuls of dark green leafy vegetables every day.
- Have an Epsom salts bath or footbath twice a week.
- Swap from white starch to brown starch, e.g. brown rice or wholemeal bread.
- Limit your consumption of fizzy drinks or sodas.
- Opt for wholefoods over processed foods, to maximize your exposure to magnesium.
- Reduce your alcohol consumption.

Energy Action Plan – my next steps

What can you do to support your magnesium levels, if you think it's a potential concern for you? Could you add more leafy greens to your diet? Would an Epsom salts bath help you unwind? Make a note of whatever stood out to you in this section and create a commitment to tackling the issue. Increasing magnesium levels can be a gamechanger for your energy and overall wellbeing!

Focus on these three questions to create your SMART objectives:

1. What will I do?
2. How will I do it?
3. When will I do it by?

YOUR GUIDE TO VITAMIN D

Quiz 6 (see page 110) highlighted some of the common symptoms of vitamin D deficiency. Read on to find out more about how this might be affecting you and your energy levels.

Vitamin D is a nutrient that actually behaves rather like a hormone, and it has multiple roles in the body. It's so important to our health and wellbeing that Mother Nature hasn't left it up to us and our erratic diets to get what we need. In fact, it's only found in food in very small quantities.

We get the bulk of our vitamin D through exposure to sunlight. It comes in two forms: ergocalciferol or vitamin D2, which comes from plants; and cholecalciferol or vitamin D3, which comes from animal sources or via the action of the sun's UVB rays on the skin. Vitamin D3 is more bioavailable and more easily absorbed by the body than D2, making it the preferred form for supplementation.

Whether we access vitamin D through food, supplements or sunlight, it always needs to be converted to the active form of vitamin D. This process takes place in the liver and kidneys.

Vitamin D has multiple roles in the body. It's perhaps best known for ensuring healthy bones and teeth, because of the part it plays in calcium absorption and supporting bone mineralization, which reduces the risk of osteoporosis.

It's also very important for our immune function, and underpins the innate immune system, which is the body's first line of defence against infection. Studies have shown that there may be an association between vitamin D deficiency and the severity and longevity of Covid-19 symptoms.

How does vitamin D support my energy levels?

There is an increasing body of research around the broad range of benefits from optimal vitamin D levels. For example, we need this vitamin to support the function of the thyroid gland, which is important for our energy levels.

Vitamin D is important for mood and mental health as well. A deficiency may well be a factor in Seasonal Affective Disorder (the winter blues) and could contribute to symptoms of depression and anxiety. This is because the sun's UVB rays are too weak during the wintertime for us to synthesize vitamin D through exposure to sunlight.

Vitamin D supports the effective functioning of mitochondria in the cells, as part of the energy production process. We also need it to produce serotonin in the brain, which helps to promote positive mood and motivation.

It's a hugely important nutrient for our health and wellbeing, and yet low levels of vitamin D are incredibly common across the general population, particularly during the winter months. This is especially true of those who are housebound, who cover up in the sun, and for people of Asian or African ethnicity, who will be more predisposed to vitamin D deficiency.

A study in 2022 by the Office for Health Improvement and Disparities (OHID) in the UK showed that 1 in 6 adults were deficient in vitamin D. In the USA, the National Health and Nutrition Examination Survey (NHANES) in 2021 suggested that 35 per cent of adults had insufficient levels.

Typical signs of vitamin D deficiency

- Bone pain
- Aching joints
- Muscle weakness
- Back pain, low energy
- Unexplained fatigue

- Insomnia
- Seasonal Affective Disorder
- Frequent colds and infections
- Dental issues

Why might the menopause affect my vitamin D levels?

As we progress through the menopause, there is an increased risk of elevated cholesterol and coronary heart disease, due to the drop in the protective effects of oestrogen on the heart muscle. Some women also struggle with menopausal weight gain.

In either case, this may encourage you to follow a very low-fat diet. This could directly affect your levels of vitamin D, because it's a fat-soluble vitamin, which means that the body stores it in fat cells for use when we need it.

The winter blues

From October to March, the UVB rays in the northern hemisphere are too weak to synthesize vitamin D, even on a nice sunny day. This can contribute to people experiencing a low mood in these months.

There is also an increasing trend toward following a largely plant-based diet. While vitamin D is only found in food in small amounts, its main sources are animal products, so being a vegan may further contribute to lower levels of this important nutrient.

We're more likely to use a high-factor sunscreen at this stage of life, to protect our skin from the ageing effects of sun damage. This will affect our ability to produce vitamin D through exposure to sunlight.

Potential causes of vitamin D depletion

- Lack of exposure to sunlight if you're housebound or tend to cover up outside
- It's wintertime – your vitamin D stores have run out
- Consistent use of high-factor sunscreen
- Having a darker skin pigment, making you more predisposed to vitamin D deficiency
- Getting older, which makes your ability to convert and absorb vitamin D from sunlight less efficient
- Following a vegan diet and avoiding exposure to sunshine
- A very low-fat diet, which can impair vitamin D absorption
- The use of certain medications, which can impair vitamin D absorption
- Chronic liver or kidney conditions, which can disrupt vitamin D metabolism

UNDERSTANDING YOUR TEST RESULTS

If you experience any of the deficiency symptoms listed above, you should consult your doctor to request a blood test to assess your vitamin D status.

The most reliable marker of vitamin D is serum 25-hydroxyvitamin D concentration, also known as serum 25(OH)D, which is how it may appear on your test results. This is considered the gold standard approach to testing, because it reflects overall vitamin D status from all potential sources.

Your results are likely to be measured in either nanomoles per litre (nmol/L) or nanograms per millilitre (ng/mL), depending on the preference of the laboratory.

Reference Ranges	Vitamin D Status
<30nmol/L or <12ng/mL	Severe deficiency
30–50nmol/L or 12–20ng/mL	Moderate deficiency
50–75nmol/L or 20–30ng/mL	Insufficient to adequate
>75nmol/L or >30ng/mL	Optimal
>250nmol/L or >100ng/mL	Potential toxicity

If your score is less than 50nmol/L or 20ng/mL, your doctor is likely to prescribe vitamin D3 supplements to correct the deficiency. They may consider anything over 50nmol/L or 20ng/mL to be adequate and may not prescribe a therapeutic dose. However, optimal levels of vitamin D would require a result higher than 75nmol/L or 30ng/mL. This would support strong bones, a healthy immune function, and physical and mental energy. It would also help to rule out any of the niggling symptoms associated with low levels of vitamin D.

Excessive blood levels of vitamin D (i.e. greater than 250nmol/L or 100ng/mL) are unusual, as this would require enormously high daily doses over a considerable period of time. However, if this is the case, you should speak to your doctor urgently so that they can take the appropriate action to address the risk of toxicity.

DIETARY SOURCES OF VITAMIN D

There are very few foods that contain more than traces of vitamin D. The foods in the table below are the richest sources of vitamin D, and even then, you can see that the amounts are relatively minimal. You would need to be eating impossibly large quantities of these foods every day to get anywhere near the recommended adult daily dose of 1,000IU of vitamin D3.

Vitamin D3 supplements are usually measured in international units (IU), rather than milligrams or micrograms. This reflects the amount of active vitamin D available. For example, 10 micrograms is equivalent to 400IU.

VITAMIN D CONTENT OF EVERYDAY FOODS PER 100G (OR AS STATED)

Wild salmon 9mcg/360IU

Mackerel 8mcg/320IU

Sardines 4mcg/160IU

1 egg yolk 3mcg/120IU

UV-exposed mushrooms* 3mcg/120IU

Fortified breakfast cereal (per 30g portion) 2mcg/80IU

Fortified cow's milk 1mcg/40IU

Liver 1mcg/40IU

*These are mushrooms that have been exposed to UV light which increases their vitamin D2 content. They can be found in supermarkets and are sometimes called vitamin D mushrooms.

EXAMPLES OF FOOD THAT CONTAIN SOME VITAMIN D

Breakfast	Lunch	Dinner	Snacks
2 poached eggs with wholemeal toast	Sardine fish cakes with salad, and a dash of mayonnaise	UV mushroom omelette	Smoked mackerel or homemade UV mushroom pâté with 1–2 oatcakes
Fortified breakfast cereal with cow's milk or plant-based milk	UV mushroom risotto	Grilled salmon with mixed vegetables	A boiled egg with spinach leaves

Vitamin D supplements

If you're already taking a multivitamin and mineral supplement, it's likely to contain vitamin D3 at a dosage of 400IU or 10mcg (or occasionally expressed as 10µg). This is a relatively low dose, more suitable for children, and you may benefit from a higher amount. A separate vitamin D3 supplement would be more appropriate than doubling the dose in your multivitamin, ensuring that you avoid unnecessarily high levels of other nutrients in the product.

I believe that a daily vitamin D3 supplement is essential for women throughout mid- and later life, even during the summer months. While you may opt for a lower dose during this time, depending on your sun exposure, it's important to ensure you maintain adequate levels year-round.

Our risk of osteoporosis increases significantly as we move through and beyond menopause, making it crucial to support optimal bone density. Taking a vitamin D3 supplement is a simple way to achieve this, as we need sufficient levels of this vitamin to absorb the calcium we consume through diet or supplements. Calcium is essential for maintaining strong, healthy bones and reducing the risk of fractures from falls or bumps.

Choosing the right vitamin D supplement & dosage

If your blood test reveals low or suboptimal levels of vitamin D, it's important to take a supplement, especially if you experience any of the symptoms associated with deficiency or are at a higher risk. I recommend a vitamin D3 (cholecalciferol) supplement, as it is typically more effectively absorbed than vitamin D2. You can take vitamin D3 in various forms – tablets, oral sprays or drops mixed with water – depending on your preference.

For optimal maintenance, a daily dosage for an adult typically ranges between 1,000IU and 3,000IU. If your blood tests indicate a deficiency, your doctor may recommend a higher therapeutic dose for a short period before retesting to evaluate your vitamin D levels.

When supplementing independently, especially if you're using home test kits, it's important not to exceed 4,000IU daily to avoid the risk of toxicity. Be sure to check all the supplements you're taking, as products like fish oils, bone complexes, and other multi-nutrient formulas may also contain vitamin D3, which can quickly add up.

CASE STUDY: Restoring vitality with vitamin D – Sophie's story

Sophie, 45, came to see me feeling sluggish, struggling with frequent colds, and dealing with achy muscles and back pain. She assumed these symptoms were just part of getting older, but after exploring her lifestyle, I discovered that Sophie worked indoors and rarely got outside in the sunlight, and it became clear that her vitamin D levels might be a concern. A blood test confirmed her levels were low. I recommended a high-quality vitamin D supplement, along with dietary adjustments to include foods that support vitamin D levels, such as oily fish, fortified foods and egg yolks. Sophie also started spending more time outdoors each day. Within a few weeks of starting the supplement and adjusting her lifestyle, Sophie reported feeling much more energetic, with fewer aches and pains. Her mood improved, and she was back to enjoying her daily activities without feeling drained.

Easy ways to boost your vitamin D levels

- Spend time outside in the spring and summer months to build up your stores for the winter. Doing this for 10–15 minutes daily should suffice to ensure you get the vitamin D you need without putting your skin at risk of sunburn. You know your skin best, so do what feels right for you.
- Include eggs, oily fish or UV mushrooms in your diet three times per week.
- Take 1,000–3,000IU of vitamin D3 every day, according to your requirements.

Energy Action Plan – my next steps

What are you going to do to support your vitamin D levels? This might involve speaking to your doctor to arrange a test. Do you need to get outside more? Should you start taking a supplement?

This is where your beautiful notebook comes in! Make a note of whatever stood out to you in this section and create a commitment to tackling the issue.

Focus on these three questions to create your SMART objectives:

1. What will I do?
2. How will I do it?
3. When will I do it by?

UNDERSTANDING A FOOD SENSITIVITY

Quiz 7 (see page 111) covers an area that is very common but is often overlooked. If the list of symptoms in this quiz included issues that you experience, it's worth considering whether one or more foods may be contributing to your fatigue.

An undiagnosed food sensitivity will lead to a state of chronic low-grade inflammation, which will have a direct impact on your energy levels (we explore this issue in more detail in Step 5, see page 266). It may also affect your ability to absorb nutrients that are essential for the body's energy production process.

The symptoms of a food intolerance or allergy can be many and varied, and different people experience them in different ways. Some people might experience digestive difficulties while others might have skin problems or headaches. Sometimes the symptoms can be quite random or unexpected, such as joint pain or difficulty in losing weight.

How does a food sensitivity affect my energy levels?

Fatigue is a common symptom of food sensitivity, often experienced as feelings of sluggishness or tiredness, or even post-meal crashes. For some individuals, it may impact mental clarity, leading to issues such as brain fog or cognitive difficulties. Many people report a noticeable shift in mental acuity – feeling sharper or more focused – after eliminating trigger foods from their diet. As the experience of food sensitivity is highly individual, treatment requires a tailored and personal approach.

Typical signs of a food sensitivity

- Fatigue or lethargy
- Brain fog
- Bloating or flatulence
- Loose stools
- Diarrhoea or constipation
- Hives
- Eczema, psoriasis, dermatitis
- Rosacea or acne
- Headaches
- Sinusitis, rhinitis, post-nasal drip
- Joint pain
- Palpitations

What is a food sensitivity?

Food intolerances or allergies are generated by the immune system. If it mistakenly perceives a food as a harmful pathogen (such as the virus causing measles or pneumonia, for example), it will trigger an antibody reaction as a protective response. This causes inflammation, which, in excess, can lead to any of the symptoms set out above.

Allergies and intolerances are not the same thing. The allergy antibody is immunoglobulin E (IgE) and the intolerance antibody is immunoglobulin G (IgG). It's perfectly possible to be allergic but not intolerant to something, or the reverse. They are distinct and separate reactions, even if they might generate many of the same symptoms.

Although it's quite common to have a very mild allergy, which may only cause minor symptoms from the list above, an excessive IgE allergic reaction may lead to an anaphylactic reaction. This is where swelling occurs in the mouth, throat or lungs that can impair your breathing and may be life-threatening.

If you have an allergy, you should always discuss it with your doctor, so that they can advise on the need for carrying an EpiPen in case of emergency. An EpiPen is a simple mechanism for injecting adrenaline (known as epinephrine in the USA) into the system to open up the airways in the case of an anaphylactic reaction.

Aside from that, the main difference between an IgE allergy and an IgG intolerance is the speed of reaction. With an allergy, any symptoms will come on very quickly, usually within an hour.

An intolerance could also manifest that quickly, or it could take up to 72 hours for symptoms to show. As a result, it's often a lot harder to identify a food intolerance than it is a food allergy.

People who have some form of food allergy often have an instinct about it. If you vomit every time you eat an apple, for example, it doesn't take long to join the dots!

Unexpectedly developing food sensitivities

A food sensitivity can pop up at any time in life. It's not necessarily something that you're born with, and developing one at some point in adulthood is quite common.

Could my menopause trigger a food sensitivity?

There is little research into this issue at present, however it's not uncommon for women to develop a food sensitivity as they transition through menopause.

One possible reason for this is the change in hormone levels that can affect the balance of the microbiota in the gut, that lovely garden of beneficial bacteria that support our health and wellbeing in a multitude of ways.

The correct balance of gut bacteria is required to support optimal digestive function, stool formation and nutrient absorption. It's also very important for a healthy immune system. Over 70 per cent of our immune cells are in the gut wall and they rely on our beneficial bacteria to work well. Dysbiosis, which is an imbalance between the so-called friendly and unfriendly bacteria, can disrupt the immune function, triggering an abnormal antibody reaction, which may lead to a food sensitivity.

Other common causes of dysbiosis include antibiotic use, bacterial infection in the gut, stress, and a low-fibre or a high-sugar diet. Certain prescription medication or medical treatments may also disrupt the bacterial balance.

How do I identify a food sensitivity?

The gold standard approach to identifying a food sensitivity is to keep a food diary to help pick up any patterns that might indicate a trigger food, and then to eliminate the food for a period to assess any symptoms.

If you already have a suspicion about a food, then it's wise to start with that, because the chances are that your instinct is right. This could save you a lot of time.

If your symptoms happen every single day, it's worth looking at some of the foods that feature daily. It's possible to be allergic or intolerant to anything, but some of the most common food sensitivities relate to dairy, yeast, eggs, and wheat or gluten. Avoiding one or more of these everyday food groups might make the world of difference to how you feel.

If you suspect an IgE food allergy, you should speak to your doctor about it to get the correct long-term advice and support, especially if your symptoms relate to any form of oral swelling or inflammation.

An IgG food intolerance can often be reversed after a strict period of elimination. The recommended approach would be 12 weeks, which research suggests is the minimum time needed for the overreacting antibodies to calm down. Once the immune system has had an opportunity to reset itself, you may be able to reintroduce the food.

Coeliac disease

Gluten intolerance is always a symptom of the autoimmune condition coeliac disease. You can be intolerant to gluten without having coeliac disease, but you can't have coeliac disease without also being gluten intolerant.

Testing for food intolerance and allergies

Testing could be a quicker route for you, if you're struggling to identify which food might be a trigger for your symptoms. An IgE allergy test will be available from your doctor, usually in the form of a skin patch test or a blood test.

IgG intolerance tests, on the other hand, are rarely available from your doctor, although there are multiple options online. The only evidence-based test for IgG antibodies is a blood test. There is no scientific evidence to support hair testing or electromagnetic testing for food intolerances.

Before investing in an online blood test, I'd recommend ensuring that the laboratory you choose has a stringent quality control system and that they are open about their compliance with the regulations in place for these tests. Look for labs that are accredited and transparent about their testing methods and quality control practices.

MANAGING AN ELIMINATION DIET FOR AN IGG FOOD INTOLERANCE

Once you've identified the food that you want to eliminate, these are the steps to take:

1. Eliminate the food completely from your diet for at least 12 weeks. Avoid all forms of the food, including where it features as an ingredient.
2. If you suspect, or if your test results show, that you are intolerant to more than one thing, it's fine to eliminate a couple of food groups, so long as you maintain a balanced diet by using sensible alternatives.
3. Unless you have a severe allergy, don't worry about a label that says "may contain traces of". This is just to flag up the potential of cross-contamination in the factory.
4. Keep a food and symptom diary to track any improvements.
5. Many free-from foods can be quite expensive and they're often very processed. You may find it cheaper and healthier simply to cook from scratch using wholefoods and ingredients that naturally don't contain that food, rather than a manufactured imitation.
6. Don't worry if there's the odd lapse. That's life. However, it is important to be as strict as possible, so that the antibodies can settle down. This will give you a greater chance to reintroduce the food after the 12-week elimination.

Here are some common trigger foods to consider eliminating.

Wheat or gluten

Wheat and gluten are not the same thing. When you are intolerant or allergic to something, it is the protein in the food that your antibodies are reacting to. Gluten is a protein found in wheat, rye and barley, but these foods also include other proteins that you might react to, so it is possible to be intolerant to wheat and not to gluten, for example.

Foods commonly containing wheat or gluten	Possible alternatives
Bread and bread products, including pizza bases, croissants, crumpets, bagels and flatbreads	Gluten-free bread is generally also wheat-free, so this can be a good option. Rye bread could be a good choice if your issue is wheat and not gluten. Some studies have also shown that the lengthy fermentation process used for making genuine sourdough bread can pre-digest the wheat and the gluten, making it less reactive for people with non-coeliac-related gluten and wheat sensitivities.
Biscuits, pastries, cakes and other baked products	Opt for oat-based biscuits. Try gluten-free baked products.
Anything with a pie or pastry crust	Keep an eye out for gluten-free alternatives, or use a gluten-free flour to make your own pastry.
Pasta and noodles	Try wheat-free pasta, which is easily available. Use a different form of starch, such as rice, quinoa, corn or polenta, buckwheat or potatoes. These are all naturally gluten and wheat-free.

Foods commonly containing wheat or gluten	Possible alternatives
Breakfast cereals	Opt for oat-based products, such as muesli, granola, porridge or oatmeal. Oats do not contain gluten, so cross-contamination is only a consideration if you have coeliac disease.
Beer or lager	Gluten-free beers, cider, wine
Soy sauce	Use tamari instead, which is a gluten-free soy sauce.

Dairy products

A true dairy intolerance is a reaction to cow's milk protein. Lactose intolerance is not the same thing. Lactose is a sugar found in milk. Some people don't produce an enzyme that breaks down lactose in the gut, which can cause unpleasant digestive problems. A lactose intolerance will not generate the other common symptoms of a food intolerance, because it's purely a mechanical digestive issue. It is usually diagnosed via a breath test that you can get from your doctor.

There are two principal proteins found in cow's milk: A1 and A2. A2 protein is also present in goat's and sheep's milk, but A1 is not. If you are only intolerant to A1 protein, you may still be able to consume goat's and sheep's milk products, giving you more flexibility during an elimination diet. However, if you are intolerant to A2 protein, you will need to avoid all dairy products containing A2 protein.

Many plant-based milks are fortified with calcium, if you're concerned that eliminating dairy might affect your calcium status. Dark green leafy vegetables and broccoli are also a very good source of calcium. Canned salmon and sardines contain plenty of calcium too, due to the soft bones.

Foods commonly containing dairy	Possible alternatives
Milk and cream	Soya, almond, oat, coconut or other plant-based milks. Consider goat's milk, if you think you can tolerate the A2 protein.
Butter	Olive or sunflower oil spreads
Yogurt	Alternative yogurts, such as soya, coconut or oat milk products. Sheep's or goat's yogurt is available in supermarkets for an A2 option.
Cheese	Opt for a plant-based cheese. A2 options (made with sheep's or goat's milk) include goat's cheese, manchego, roquefort or pecorino. Traditionally, feta cheese and halloumi are made with only sheep's or goat's milk, meaning they contain A2 protein. However, some supermarkets blend them with cow's milk to reduce costs, so it's important to check the label carefully before purchasing.
Baked products, cakes, desserts, ice cream, products made with batter, chocolate	Opt for plant-based options of these foods. There are plenty of good products available or recipes online if you want to make your own.

Eggs

An egg intolerance is often overlooked, but it's something I frequently encounter in my nutrition clinic. More commonly, people are intolerant to egg whites, but in some cases, the yolk can cause issues too.

Foods commonly containing eggs	Possible alternatives
Any form of egg, e.g. poached egg, boiled egg, scrambled egg	Swap to a different breakfast, e.g overnight oats; or avocado and smoked salmon on toast.
Cakes and baked products	Use aquafaba or chickpea/garbanzo bean water as an alternative for egg when baking
Batter mixes, e.g. pancakes, Yorkshire pudding, battered fish	Opt for a vegan product or try an egg replacement powder if you're making your own.
Quiche or frittata	Try a vegetable-based tart instead.
Some gluten-free breads	Check the label carefully for egg white, which is a common addition in some brands, and opt for an egg-free product.
Chocolate mousse, meringue, custard, marshmallows and most baked desserts	Opt for vegan products; check out aquafaba or chickpea/garbanzo bean water as a raising agent in a recipe, or to make meringues.
Mayonnaise, salad cream, Béarnaise or Hollandaise sauces	There are lots of good vegan versions of these products in supermarkets.

Foods commonly containing eggs	Possible alternatives
Burgers, veggie burgers and meatballs, which may be bound with egg	Check labels or menus carefully for allergy advice, and select an egg-free product.
Breaded meat or fish, which may be dipped in egg to make the breadcrumbs stick	Check labels or menus carefully for allergy advice, and select an egg-free product.

Yeast

A yeast sensitivity is something I have observed more frequently in my nutrition clinic in recent years. People who have reactions to bread and beer often assume it's the wheat or gluten, but if eliminating either of these brings no relief, it could be worth considering yeast as a potential factor.

Eliminating yeast from your diet can be tricky because it's found in many foods, and natural yeast, which is present in the air and on surfaces, can settle on a variety of foods. This means even foods that don't have yeast added can sometimes contain small amounts. However, by cutting out the most common sources of yeast, you can still make a big difference in how you feel.

There is often some confusion online regarding yeast sensitivities. It is important to note that this is not the same as an overgrowth of candida in the gut. While both can coexist, they are distinct issues – candida overgrowth is typically diagnosed through a stool test. Advice surrounding a low-sugar diet, which is usually supervised by a health professional, is specific to candida management and does not directly apply to managing a yeast intolerance.

Foods commonly containing yeast	Possible alternatives
Bread and bread products, e.g. pizza bases, Danish pastries and croissants, crumpets, bagels and certain flatbreads such as pitta or naan bread	Soda bread is made with bicarbonate of soda and not yeast. Genuine sourdough is made without added baker's yeast, drawing instead on the natural yeast in the environment as a raising agent (but do check the label, because sourdough is not a protected term and some products may still contain yeast).
Yeast extract spreads; nutritional yeast	Check labels carefully for yeast extract and use alternative flavourings, such as sundried tomatoes or liquid aminos (see below).
Fermented health foods, such as kefir, kimchi, sauerkraut and kombucha	Natural yogurt is usually fine, because it is far less fermented than kefir.
Fermented condiments such as soy sauce or all vinegars, including malt, wine, apple cider, balsamic or rice vinegars	Liquid aminos are an unfermented soy sauce. Spirit vinegar, which is distilled and not fermented, is used in some pickles and other condiments, such as mayonnaise or ketchup. Check the labels to be sure.
Fermented alcohol: all beer, wine, cider, rum	Gin, vodka, tequila and some malt whiskies are distilled. Champagne is sufficiently filtered to remove yeast (this does not apply to Prosecco, cava or other sparkling wines).

Foods commonly containing yeast	Possible alternatives
Mushrooms and mushroom-based vegetarian products, e.g. myco protein	Check labels carefully to avoid any mushrooms and opt for aubergine/eggplant, fennel or artichoke hearts to replace mushrooms in your recipes.

How to manage reintroduction after 12 weeks

At the end of your 12-week elimination period, it's time to reintroduce the foods to see how you react. It's important to be systematic about this process and keep a notebook or spreadsheet to track your progress and symptoms as you gradually reintroduce the foods one by one. Treat it like a scientific experiment: only change one thing at a time to clearly identify any problematic reactions. These are the steps to follow:

1. **Choose a form of the food** you want to reintroduce (e.g. if you eliminated all dairy, choose milk, cheese or yogurt; if you avoided wheat, select bread, pasta or cereal). Consistency is key – once you decide on the form of food you are reintroducing, stick to it.

2. **Week 1:** Introduce a standard portion of the food on your chosen day (e.g. cheese on a Friday), and observe your reaction over the coming days. If you experience any reaction – whether it's fatigue, digestive issues or another symptom – discontinue the food for another 12 weeks before trying again.

3. **Week 2:** If there were no issues, introduce another standard portion of the food twice in the second week (e.g. Friday and Tuesday), and continue to monitor your symptoms.

4. **Week 3:** If you still experience no problems, introduce the food three times in the third week (e.g. Friday, Monday and Wednesday).

5. Gradually build it up each week to assess your tolerance and symptoms.

6. If you experience any issues at any point, discontinue the food and note when you stopped. You may find that you can tolerate small amounts periodically.

7. You may wish to stop at Week 3 and try a different form of the food, such as switching from cheese to yogurt if you started with cheese.

8. After reintroduction, one of three things will happen:
   a). You'll be fine with that food now and can consume it regularly.
   b). The food is okay in small doses or specific forms, but frequent consumption might cause issues.
   c). You feel better avoiding it altogether, so you'll need to avoid it entirely to manage symptoms.

9. Each time you change the form of food you're testing, allow at least three days between reintroductions to ensure that it's clear what may have caused any reactions.

10. If you do experience symptoms, wait until you've had three to four symptom-free days before trialling another food.

11. It's not uncommon to tolerate a food in one form but not another. For example, some may manage cheese or yogurt but struggle with milk or cream, or cope with baker's yeast but not brewer's yeast. Different processing methods or forms of a food may be more or less problematic.

12. Don't be discouraged if the reintroduction doesn't work immediately. Sometimes, the immune system simply needs more time to settle, and longer elimination phases may be required. In other cases, avoiding the food altogether may yield the best results. Everyone's experience is unique.

Easy ways to manage an elimination diet

- Keep a diary to score the severity of your symptoms as you go along. This will help you track your progress. As you start to feel better, it can be easy to forget how you felt before.
- If you find the idea of a full 12 weeks daunting, start with a strict two-week elimination. That should be enough to give you an idea of the impact on your energy levels or other symptoms. If you experience a significant improvement, you'll be more motivated to continue for the remaining ten weeks.
- Cook meals from scratch, so that you are in control of the ingredients.
- When eating out, check the menu online for allergen information or phone the restaurant in advance, to avoid awkwardness when you order your food. The staff are generally very happy to oblige, because some advance warning makes it easier for the kitchen.
- Prepare a packed lunch or suitable snacks for when you're on the go. It can be very hard to find the right foods if options are limited.
- Identify treats that you like and that work for you in advance. Twelve weeks is a long time and it's much better to know how to indulge wisely than to assume you won't have a sugary snack or alcoholic drink for the whole period. That way you won't undo all your good work.

CASE STUDY: Restoring balance and vitality with an elimination diet – Rachel's story

Rachel, 40, came to see me after struggling with bloating, digestive discomfort and low energy. She'd already ruled out any medical condition, but she was no further forward. After a detailed discussion about her symptoms and diet, I suspected a food sensitivity might be at play. We decided to explore this further through an elimination diet, removing common culprits such as dairy and gluten as a first step. After a few weeks, Rachel noticed significant improvement in her digestion and energy. To pinpoint the specific trigger, we gradually reintroduced foods back into her diet. She discovered that dairy was the main culprit behind her discomfort, and she continued to avoid it for three months. Over this time, Rachel's digestion improved, and she felt much lighter and more energetic. She was relieved to have finally figured out what was causing her symptoms and now felt in control of her health.

Energy Action Plan – my next steps

What changes could you make if you suspect a food sensitivity? Do you need to speak to your doctor? If you already suspect a food sensitivity, is it time to take the plunge and follow an elimination diet for 12 weeks? Might you benefit from a food intolerance test?

Make a note of whatever stood out to you in this section and create a commitment to tackling the issue

Focus on these three questions to create your SMART objectives:

1. What will I do?
2. How will I do it?
3. When will I do it by?

Building on your progress

Over the past two chapters, we've delved into the different ways that your diet can influence energy levels. You've come to understand the importance of a balanced intake of macronutrients, and I hope you've already noticed some positive changes from your 14-Day Energy Boost Programme. You should also now feel more confident in identifying and addressing any micronutrient or functional imbalances in your body.

In the next phase of our journey, we'll shift focus to lifestyle factors and how they impact your energy. Let's move on to Step 5 of your journey through The Happy Menopause Energy Clinic to delve into the various elements that may be contributing to your sense of fatigue.

STEP 5

ENERGY GAIN OR ENERGY DRAIN? MAKE LIFESTYLE CHOICES TO IMPROVE YOUR VITALITY

Achieving optimal energy is like completing a jigsaw puzzle: each piece is essential to create the full picture. With only some pieces there, you might glimpse the overall image, but when every piece is in place, it all fits together perfectly and your energy flows like a well-oiled machine.

We've already seen the importance of keeping on top of essential health checks (Step 2), achieving the correct balance of macronutrients (Step 3) and addressing any micronutrient or functional imbalances (Step 5). In this step of your journey though The Happy Menopause Energy Clinic, we look for the final pieces in the vitality jigsaw, examining the different lifestyle factors that can affect your energy and how smart choices can make a world of difference to the way you feel.

CAFFEINE

Caffeine is a powerful natural stimulant which, for many of us, is a regular fixture in our daily routine. A cup of tea or coffee often provides the excuse for a break, can be a reward for completing a task, or a comfort when things become difficult. It may be hard to imagine the day without tea or coffee, and the mere idea of giving up caffeine may make you feel quite anxious.

To understand why we feel so deeply attached to caffeine, it's helpful to explore the impact it has on our brain and the delicate balance of our neurotransmitters.

Caffeine's chain reaction – what happens in your brain

Caffeine acts by blocking the action of a chemical called adenosine, which builds up in the brain over the course of the day and plays a key role in the sleep–wake cycle, due to its action in slowing the brain down and activating drowsiness.

When the adenosine receptors are blocked, the brain becomes more active, creating a domino effect that sends a ripple across the brain and triggers an emergency fight-or-flight response. This leads to the release of the neurotransmitters adrenaline and noradrenaline, which increase mental alertness and wakefulness, and speed up the heart rate. This is the familiar short-term energy boost you'll experience with caffeine.

In parallel to this, the inhibitory effect of caffeine on adenosine increases levels of the reward neurotransmitter dopamine, which is associated with improved mood, motivation and mental clarity. This spike in dopamine signals a sense of reward to the brain, associating the caffeine with pleasure. Once you've metabolized the caffeine, however, the adenosine levels reactivate and the dopamine levels drop. This can leave a reward deficit that can trigger the urge for more caffeine, to recreate that sense of pleasure.

If you're feeling a bit crushed by this, don't panic! The occasional cup of tea or coffee during the day, as part of a balanced diet, should be fine. It's unlikely to overstimulate the dopamine pathways or lead to over-dependence. As with most things, moderation is key.

There are even some potential health benefits to caffeine. For example, studies have shown that it can enhance physical performance in endurance activities and help with short-term memory. Moderate tea or coffee consumption may also be linked to a reduced risk of chronic conditions, such as Parkinson's disease.

How does caffeine affect my energy levels?

If you're fond of a daily caffeine fix, a bit of a balancing act is required when it comes to energy. As we have seen above, caffeine can provide a short-term energy boost, which can be very handy at times. However, this energy boost comes with trade-offs. If you're in the habit of having several cups of tea or coffee every day, there's no doubt that this will lead to a net loss in energy. Overuse of caffeine can lead to energy crashes when the adrenaline, noradrenaline and dopamine subside, and the adenosine receptors start to function properly again. This form of rebound fatigue is especially common if you've been using caffeine to manage sleep deprivation or exhaustion.

Caffeine vs sleep: how it disturbs your rest

Caffeine is a powerful sleep disrupter. We've seen the impact it has on the adenosine receptors which influence our sleep–wake cycle. This can delay the onset of sleepiness, so that you go to bed later or take much longer to fall asleep, even if you're feeling very tired. When you've got a busy day ahead, this can be extremely stressful.

Excessive levels of caffeine will also affect the quality of sleep by impacting our sleep cycles. These cycles run in periods of 90 minutes over the course of the night, and we need to complete a number of these to achieve the full benefit of a restorative sleep. Lingering levels of caffeine in the body can cause you to wake up during the night, preventing you from completing full sleep cycles, which will leave you feeling tired and unrefreshed in the morning.

Caffeine & the mitochondria

Moderate caffeine consumption is unlikely to disrupt and may even support mitochondrial function, but too much can increase oxidative stress. This can damage the membrane of the mitochondria and impair their ability to produce energy.

Typical signs of too much caffeine

- Insomnia
- Feeling jittery or nervous
- Palpitations
- Increased heart rate
- High blood pressure
- Feeling "wired"
- Anxiety or irritability
- Headaches
- Frequent urination
- PMS
- Twitching muscles
- Caffeine crashes

How does caffeine affect my menopause?

Our ability to metabolize caffeine effectively may be affected by the decline in oestrogen, so women often become more sensitive to it during and post-menopause, and the disruptive effects of caffeine can be far-reaching. Here are some of the more common menopause symptoms that can be associated with too much caffeine.

- **Hot flushes & night sweats:** Caffeine is a well-known trigger for hot flushes and night sweats, its impact on the heart rate and blood pressure aggravating these symptoms. If you're experiencing regular problems with flushes and sweats, a simple solution could be to reduce or eliminate caffeine from your diet and see what difference that makes.

- **Nervousness & anxiety:** The emotional and psychological symptoms of the menopause, such as feeling nervous or jittery, will all be exacerbated by too much caffeine. The impact of caffeine on the central nervous system may also worsen symptoms of anxiety.

- **Mood swings:** Caffeine can also affect your mood. Although it may provide a useful short-term energy boost, as the impact wears off and the dopamine levels fall, you may find that this increases problems with mood swings.

- **Insomnia:** This can be a very real issue during the menopause, even if you're not prone to night sweats, with random hormonal surges during the night causing you to wake up frequently. Adding the sleep-disrupting impact of caffeine into the mix could simply make everything much worse.

- **Bone health:** Too much caffeine can affect calcium absorption at the very stage of life when we need optimal levels to support our bone density.

- **Heart health:** Caffeine can impact our heart health by increasing heart rate and triggering palpitations. It's also a common culprit in high blood pressure, which is a concern because women are more susceptible to hypertension post-menopause.

How does the body metabolize caffeine?

When we have a cup of tea or coffee, the effects are felt relatively quickly. Caffeine takes about 30–60 minutes to be absorbed through the digestive system and into the bloodstream. Once there, it is distributed throughout the body and crosses the blood–brain barrier to reach the brain, which is why it has such a significant impact on the central nervous system.

The half-life of caffeine – the time it takes for half of the caffeine to be eliminated from your system – is typically 4–6 hours, although this varies from person to person. Caffeine is broken down in the liver by a series of enzymatic reactions, primarily involving the enzyme CYP1A2.

Some people have a more active version of the CYP1A2 enzyme, which allows them to metabolize caffeine more quickly, and for them the effects of caffeine are shorter-lived. Those with a less active version of the enzyme, known as slow metabolizers, process caffeine more slowly, which means it stays in their system longer.

Fast metabolizers can often tolerate higher levels of caffeine without experiencing negative effects such as jitters, restlessness or insomnia, while slow metabolizers may be more sensitive.

What influences caffeine metabolism?

Genetics play a major role in the action of the CYP1A2 enzyme, but other factors can also affect how efficiently caffeine is metabolized:

- **Age:** Metabolism slows with age.
- **Medication:** Certain drugs can speed up or slow down caffeine breakdown.

- **Hormonal changes:** Shifts during pregnancy, menopause or with hormonal treatments (such as birth control) can influence CYP1A2 activity.

How much is too much caffeine?

The recommended maximum daily limit for caffeine for non-pregnant women is 400mg, although individual tolerance will vary from person to person, so even smaller amounts can trigger symptoms. If you're experiencing issues with low energy or insomnia, it would be wise to audit the timing and dosage of your caffeine intake over the day, because it's possible that what suited you before no longer suits you.

We mostly think of caffeine as tea or coffee, but it's also found in colas, energy drinks and chocolate. The darker the chocolate, the higher the caffeine content.

AVERAGE CAFFEINE CONTENT OF SELECTED POPULAR PRODUCTS

Product	Serving size	Average caffeine content
Coffee		
Filter coffee (small)	240ml	95mg
Filter coffee (medium)	355ml	140mg
Filter coffee (large)	475ml	190mg
Single espresso	30ml	63mg
Latte/cappuccino/flat white (small)	240ml (1 shot)	63mg

AVERAGE CAFFEINE CONTENT OF SELECTED POPULAR PRODUCTS

Product	Serving size	Average caffeine content
Latte/cappuccino/flat white (medium)	355ml (2 shots)	126mg
Latte/cappuccino/flat white (large)	475ml (3 shots)	189mg
Tea		
Black tea	240ml	40–70mg (depending on strength of infusion)
Chai latte	240ml	40–70mg (depending on strength of infusion)
Matcha green tea	240ml	50–70mg (depending on amount of powder used)
Green tea	240ml	20–45mg (depending on strength of infusion)
Carbonated drinks		
Cola	330ml can	33mg
Diet cola	330ml can	46mg
Energy drink	250ml can	80mg
Chocolate		
Milk chocolate	100g	15–20mg

AVERAGE CAFFEINE CONTENT OF SELECTED POPULAR PRODUCTS

Product	Serving size	Average caffeine content
70% dark chocolate	100g	70–85mg
80% dark chocolate	100g	90–100mg
90% dark chocolate	100g	110–120mg

Do you need to audit your caffeine intake?

It can be helpful to track your consumption of caffeinated foods and beverages over the course of a week. You might discover that you're consuming more caffeine than you realize, or that you're having too much of it later in the day, which could be impacting your sleep.

If you feel the need to reduce your caffeine intake, it's best to do so gradually over several days. Abruptly cutting out caffeine can lead to unpleasant withdrawal symptoms, including headaches, fatigue and irritability. The sudden change may also temporarily disrupt your sleep patterns further.

Over-reliance on caffeine affects your body's natural production of dopamine and adrenaline. By giving up caffeine gradually, your neurotransmitter receptors will reset over the course of a few days, allowing your body to produce dopamine and adrenaline naturally, without needing a caffeine boost.

Easy ways to reduce your caffeine intake

- **Order a single shot:** At the coffee shop, ask for one shot of espresso instead of two with your favourite order.
- **Use less coffee at home:** Brew with a smaller amount of ground coffee or choose a blend or pod that contains less caffeine.
- **Go half-and-half:** Mix regular coffee with decaffeinated coffee to gradually reduce your intake.
- **Brew tea for less time:** Steep your tea bag for a shorter duration to lower the caffeine content.
- **Switch to caffeine-free teas:** Experiment with caffeine-free options such as rooibos/redbush or herbal teas.
- **Choose natural decaf coffee:** Opt for decaffeinated coffee made with natural, chemical-free methods such as the Swiss Water® Process.
- **Prioritize your favourite caffeine fix:** Identify the caffeinated drink that matters most each day and stick to it, swapping the others for decaf or caffeine-free alternatives.
- **Cut caffeine after lunch:** Avoid caffeinated drinks in the afternoon to support better sleep.
- **Ditch soda and energy drinks:** Replace colas and energy drinks with sparkling water for a refreshing caffeine-free option.
- **Be cautious with dark chocolate:** Dark chocolate has some health benefits due to its antioxidants and minerals, which is a nice bonus. Opt for a couple of squares rather than a full bar, to moderate your caffeine intake.

Energy Action Plan – my next steps

Has this section given you pause for thought? If you suspect that too much caffeine might be a factor in your lack of energy, what steps could you take to address the issue? Perhaps you need to audit your caffeine intake. Have you identified some quick wins where you could easily moderate your consumption?

Make a note of whatever stood out to you in this section and create a commitment to tackling the issue.

Focus on these three questions to create your SMART objectives:

1. What will I do?
2. How will I do it?
3. When will I do it by?

ALCOHOL

What do you think of when you think about alcohol? Are you imagining enjoying a glass of fizz as part of a celebration? Do you associate it with relaxation as you curl up with a glass of wine in front of the TV? Does a quick drink help you destress after a difficult day? Is it all about a boozy evening with friends? How does alcohol fit into the patterns of your life?

It's easy to think of alcohol as an enjoyable element of our life that is very much under our control. However, recent statistics from the Institute of Alcohol Studies in the UK suggest that this may not be the case. They reveal an increasing tendency among midlife women to drink more, exacerbated during the Covid-19 pandemic, when alcohol use among women aged 30 to 64 increased by 41 per cent due to feelings of isolation and anxiety.

In the United States, a study published in *JAMA Health Forum* in 2024 found a significant rise in alcohol-related hospital admissions among middle-aged women, particularly during the pandemic, with many reporting increased alcohol use due to stress and isolation. These findings highlight that the growing pattern of alcohol misuse is affecting women across the world.

There appears to be a trend toward using alcohol as a coping mechanism for stress, with drinking behaviours influenced by pressures such as caregiving, work–life imbalance, and emotional wellbeing. The marketing of alcohol to women, which often positions it as a tool for relaxation and self-care, may have contributed to this trend.

To understand the implications of this significant shift around attitudes to alcohol, it might be helpful to understand what alcohol is and how it affects our brain and body.

What is alcohol?

When we talk about alcohol, we actually mean ethanol, which is the active ingredient in alcoholic drinks. This small molecule is classified as a depressant. It's a psychoactive substance, which means that it affects the brain and can influence our mood, perception, cognitive function and behaviour. Ethanol interacts with our central nervous system and influences the action of our neurotransmitters, the chemical messengers that regulate everything from mood and memory to reflexes and coordination.

Typical effects of alcohol consumption

- Relaxation
- Reduced anxiety
- Drowsiness
- Loss of inhibition
- Memory lapses
- Impaired judgement or decision-making
- Loss of coordination
- Slower reflexes

How does the body metabolize alcohol?

When we drink alcohol, we start absorbing it very quickly; about 20 per cent is absorbed through the stomach lining and the remainder through the small intestine. If your stomach is empty, the alcohol will be absorbed even more speedily, which is why it's not advisable to drink on an empty stomach. The presence of food will also delay the passage of alcohol into the small intestine where most of the absorption takes place.

Once the alcohol has been absorbed into the bloodstream, it will be distributed throughout the body and rapidly enter the brain, which is when the psychoactive effects will start to occur.

Alcohol is mostly metabolized through the liver, although around 10 per cent will be excreted unchanged through the skin, breath and urine. The liver will break down the alcohol through a series of enzymatic reactions, and it takes roughly an hour to break down one unit (or one standard drink of 14g – see page 227) of alcohol. If you're drinking faster than your liver can metabolize the alcohol, it will build up in the bloodstream, increasing your level of intoxication.

Risks & benefits of alcohol

The risks of excessive alcohol consumption are well documented. It's strongly associated with cardiovascular disease, liver disease and certain cancers, in particular breast, bowel, mouth and liver cancer. Alcohol weakens the immune system and can impair mood and mental health. Heavy drinking is also associated with reduced longevity.

The plus side of alcohol is less heavily weighted! As with caffeine, it's all about moderate consumption. Some studies suggest that one drink a day may reduce the risk of coronary heart disease and regulate cholesterol levels. The most effective drink is likely to be red wine, because of the resveratrol levels found in grape skins. This is a powerful antioxidant that reduces inflammation and may help to prevent damage to blood vessels. There is some research to suggest that the polyphenol content of beer may have a mildly positive impact on heart health. Spirits contain fewer antioxidants but may still provide some benefits.

However, it's very important to note that all the research on alcohol is based around one small glass daily (i.e. 150ml/5fl oz wine, half a pint of beer, a single 25ml/¾fl oz shot of spirits). Drinking more than this will not increase the benefits, and in most cases is actually likely to reverse the beneficial effect. It really is all about moderation!

How does alcohol affect my energy levels?

You might view alcohol as a bit of a pick-me-up when you're feeling tired, but the net effect on all your body systems will result in a significant energy drain on the brain and the body.

Alcohol & sleep

Alcohol acts as a sedative. Its depressant effects on the central nervous system will slow down brain activity, affecting concentration, focus and recall, and leading to fatigue and drowsiness.

Using alcohol as a nightcap may help you get off to sleep quickly, but the sedative effects will affect the quality of your sleep. Alcohol interferes with the sleep cycles, so you won't achieve the level of restorative sleep required to feel refreshed on waking and to drive your physical and mental energy levels over the course of the day.

Nutrient balance

Regular alcohol consumption affects the absorption of a number of key nutrients required for energy, in particular B vitamins and magnesium. These nutrients are crucial for the chain reaction of energy production and the formation of red blood cells required to carry oxygen around the body to support our energy.

Alcohol also interferes with blood sugar balance and will lead to an energy crash, leaving us tired, weak, irritable and unproductive (see page 113).

Alcohol is a natural diuretic which encourages the body to excrete fluid in the form of urine and this may lead to dehydration. We have already explored the impact of this on mental clarity and physical strength and stamina (see page 75).

Alcohol & the mitochondria

Ethanol disrupts the production of ATP energy molecules in the mitochondria. It also damages mitochondrial DNA, which will impair the entire energy production process, particularly in tissues that require a lot of energy, such as the brain. There will be an inevitable knock-on effect on cognitive function.

The liver is another organ with high energy demands, which is why every liver cell contains thousands of mitochondria. Excessive alcohol consumption can damage these, leading to conditions like fatty liver disease. This damage impairs the liver's ability to perform its over 500 functions, including its role in metabolizing and storing energy as glycogen for use when we need it.

Another inconvenient effect of alcohol

Anti-diuretic hormone (ADH) is released at night to reduce urine production. Alcohol blocks ADH, so if you're waking frequently to use the bathroom, it might be the alcohol, not your age!

Alcohol also increases levels of oxidative stress and inflammation, both of which will disrupt mitochondrial function.

How does alcohol affect my menopause?

As we move through perimenopause and menopause, the body copes less well with alcohol and you're likely to struggle to metabolize it effectively. There are a number of reasons for this, including the drop in oestrogen required to support alcohol metabolism in the liver, and the result may be that alcohol stays in your system for longer. This will make you more susceptible to it and more likely to experience a hangover.

Alcohol is known to trigger or exacerbate a number of common symptoms of the menopause:

- **Hot flushes and night sweats:** Alcohol is a vasodilator, which means that it expands your blood vessels which can lead to the skin flushing and sweating. Some studies have shown that regular consumption of alcohol can increase instances of hot flushes and night sweats.
- **Sleep disruption:** Alcohol disrupts sleep regardless of our age or sex, but combined with the hormonal surges that often occur, this can become much more severe during perimenopause and menopause.
- **Issues with mood and mental health:** Hormonal fluctuations during this phase of life are a common trigger for mood swings, anxiety, brain fog and loss of mental clarity. If these issues are already affecting you, they will all be significantly aggravated by alcohol.
- **Low bone density:** Regular alcohol consumption can impact bone health which is a concern during and post-menopause, as you can lose up to 25 per cent of bone density as you transition through the menopause. Alcohol blocks the absorption of the calcium we need to support strong, healthy bones, and this may increase the risk of osteopenia and osteoporosis.
- **Weight gain:** Too much alcohol is a fast route to abdominal fat and weight gain. This is already a common concern for women in midlife,

due to the changes in metabolism, and excessive levels of alcohol will exacerbate the issue.

- **Heart health:** The drop in the protective effects of oestrogen on the heart muscle can increase the risk of coronary heart disease. The role of alcohol in increasing blood pressure and cholesterol and disrupting the cardiovascular system may add to the risk of heart disease.

How much is too much alcohol?

The guideline recommended amount of alcohol for women varies slightly according to each country, although the principle of moderation remains a constant theme.

- **UK:** a maximum of 14 units spread across the week, to allow for moderation
- **USA:** up to 1 standard drink per day
- **Canada:** no more than 10 standard drinks per week, including a maximum of 3 per single day

It's important to recognize that these guidelines represent a maximum, and not a target!

I'd recommend aiming for at least four consecutive alcohol-free days each week.

While any day without alcohol offers benefits, having a block of four or more alcohol-free days gives your liver the time it needs to focus on its many essential functions, such as energy metabolism. Think of it like switching off your Wi-Fi: without incoming emails (alcohol), your system can catch up on its backlog and work more efficiently.

Here are two simple tables (one for the UK and one for North America) which set out the alcohol content of some popular drinks. You might find it helpful to use an alcohol unit calculator app, so that you can easily keep track of your consumption in relation to your local health guidelines.

UK ALCOHOL CONTENT MEASURED IN UNITS OF ALCOHOL PER MILLILITRE (ML)

Drink	Measure	Number of alcohol units
Wine (11%)	175ml	1.9
Wine (13%)	175ml	2.3
Sparkling wine (11%)	125ml	1.4
Sparkling wine (13%)	125ml	1.6
Fortified wine (20%)	50ml	1
Premium lager (5%)	1 pint	3
IPA (craft beer) (6%)	1 pint	3.4

USA & CANADA ALCOHOL CONTENT MEASURED IN STANDARD DRINKS PER FLUID OUNCE (FL OZ)

Drink	US standard drink (14g alcohol)	Canada standard drink (13.6g alcohol)
Wine (11%)	5 fl oz → 1 standard drink	5 fl oz → 1 standard drink
Wine (13%)	5 fl oz → 1 standard drink	5 fl oz → 1 standard drink
Sparkling wine (11%)	5 fl oz → 1 standard drink	5 fl oz → 1 standard drink
Sparkling wine (13%)	5 fl oz → 1 standard drink	5 fl oz → 1 standard drink

USA & CANADA ALCOHOL CONTENT MEASURED IN STANDARD DRINKS PER FLUID OUNCE (FL OZ)		
Drink	**US standard drink (14g alcohol)**	**Canada standard drink (13.6g alcohol)**
Fortified wine (20%)	1.7 fl oz → 1 standard drink	1.7 fl oz → 1 standard drink
Premium lager (5%)	12 fl oz → 1 standard drink	12 fl oz → 1 standard drink
IPA – craft beer (6%)	12 fl oz → 1.2 standard drinks	12fl oz → 1.2 standard drinks

Could you benefit from cutting back on alcohol?

When life is busy and stressful, it's easy to slide into using alcohol as a support mechanism to help you relax. We often don't realize how much alcohol is in our favourite tipple – the strength of wine or beer can vary significantly, depending on the vineyard or the brewery. You might have got into the habit of drinking a small amount every night, or perhaps you're a bit of a binge drinker when you socialize.

Use the relevant table above to assess your alcohol intake and see where you sit within the recommended guidelines. But don't forget that these are based on a broad range of people and even smaller amounts of alcohol might impact your health and wellbeing.

If you're experiencing low energy, lack of mental clarity or struggle generally with menopause symptoms, you may well benefit from taking a break altogether. A month away from alcohol could be a gamechanger for the way you feel and would allow you time to create healthy habits that would serve you well.

Easy ways to moderate your alcohol consumption

- **Smart ordering:** Order wine by the glass rather than the bottle when you eat out. This will help you keep track of the exact quantity you're consuming.
- **Use smaller glasses at home:** This will ensure you automatically serve a smaller amount.
- **Go single!** Order a single measure of spirits rather than a double when you're at a bar.
- **Be measured:** Buy a spirit measure to use at home. A single spirit measure is smaller than you might think and if you're measuring by eye, you're likely to be over-generous.
- **Use an app:** Download an alcohol unit calculator app for easy reference.
- **Take the car:** Offer to be the designated driver on a night out: it's a handy way to avoid peer pressure around drinking.
- **Be smart at the bar:** When it's your turn to buy drinks, order a sparkling water with ice and lemon – this can easily pass for a gin & tonic, if you're feeling under pressure to drink alcohol.
- **Go low!** Opt for low-alcohol beer or wine – there are lots of very good products available and this will help you keep the unit content down.
- **Research alcohol-free options:** There are some delicious choices out there – try a virgin mojito or one of the other alcohol-free cocktails, or maybe a kombucha or a Seedlip drink.
- **Change your social routines:** Meet friends for activities that don't involve alcohol: go for a walk, do a fitness class together or try out a new hobby.
- **Give your liver a break:** Aim for at least three consecutive alcohol-free days each week.

Energy Action Plan – my next steps

How do you feel about alcohol? Is it serving you well or is it time to change a few things. It's not always easy to move away from a long-standing habit, so take it a step at a time. Pick one or two areas where you feel that you could successfully make changes and build on that.

Make a note of whatever stood out to you in this section and create a commitment to supporting your physical and mental energy through moderation.

These are the three questions you need to focus on to create your SMART objectives:

1. What will I do?
2. How will I do it?
3. When will I do it by?

EXERCISE

Are you too tired to exercise? Or are you tired because you're not exercising *enough*? There's a conundrum!

If you're feeling tired all the time, exercise is often the first thing to go out the window. After all, how can you possibly find the time and energy to exercise, when you haven't the time or energy to complete all your daily tasks?

It may seem contradictory, but exercise is a crucial part of the energy equation and can perk you up considerably if you're feeling tired, jaded or lethargic. The World Health Organization recommends 300 minutes (five hours) of physical activity each week, of which 150 minutes (two and a half hours) should be vigorous exercise. That might seem like a mountain to climb if you can barely summon up the energy to get up in the morning, but it could make a material difference to your energy levels. Let's take a look at what might be holding you back.

Barriers to exercise

Statistics show that many women in midlife are very far from achieving the WHO goal. There can be a number of reasons for this:

- **Time constraints:** We midlife women are juggling multiple responsibilities, such as work, family life and caregiving. A busy or erratic schedule often means that self-care can go out of the window, and exercise is usually the first thing that gets dropped.
- **Loss of confidence:** As the perimenopause progresses, many women feel awkward, anxious or nervous. It's quite common to experience a loss of body confidence, especially if you've recently gained weight. This can create a barrier to going to the gym or attending an exercise class.

- **Health issues:** Some of the common symptoms associated with the menopause might act as a barrier to exercise. Urinary stress incontinence, when you leak a small amount of urine if you jump or run, is incredibly common and may stop you from doing your daily run or regular high-impact class. Joint pain is another common issue – after all, if it hurts to exercise, why would you do it?
- **A sedentary lifestyle:** You work at a desk, mostly at home, so there's no commute on many days and the opportunities for movement are limited. Or perhaps you drive to and from work and sit at a desk all day.
- **Lack of variety:** You do exercise regularly, but favour one type over another, so may not be getting all the potential benefits.
- **Procrastination:** You're going to start your regime on Monday. Yes, you really are! But you say that every week, and in the meantime the gym is doing very nicely out of your direct debit.
- **Fatigue:** Despite all the known benefits of exercise, it can be hard to find the motivation when all you want to do is lie down on the sofa.

Studies have shown, however, that lack of exercise might actually contribute to fatigue, and if you move more, then you're likely to experience an improvement in your daily energy levels. Let's explore the different ways that exercise can give us an energy boost: this might help to motivate you to be more active.

Common signs of lack of exercise

- Lethargy
- Loss of motivation
- Lack of muscle tone
- Low bone density
- Poor sleep
- Weight gain
- Lower back pain
- Breathless during minor exertion
- Constipation
- Consistent fatigue

How does exercise help my energy levels?

The first and most obvious way that exercise supports our energy levels is that it improves our circulation. Blood moves more efficiently around the body and the brain, and, with it, oxygen, which is one of the key ingredients in the production of energy. If there's more oxygen reaching our cells, we can produce more ATP energy molecules to power our physical and mental vitality, strength and stamina.

Exercise & the mitochondria

Regular exercise, especially endurance activities such as running, cycling or swimming, stimulates the production of new mitochondria. This creates a virtuous circle whereby exercise boosts energy production, and this in turn helps you exercise more effectively.

Physical activity optimizes mitochondrial function by enhancing the efficiency of the electron transport chain, which is responsible for generating cellular energy (see page 290). Exercise also stimulates repair processes, ensuring the mitochondria remain productive and functional as we age. And it triggers the production of antioxidants, which help to protect mitochondrial health from potentially damaging oxidative stress.

Exercise & the brain

Exercise also triggers the release of endorphins and dopamine, two neurotransmitters that have a profound impact on the brain, promoting feelings of wellbeing and reward. Endorphins are released during exercise, sex and laughter, helping to improve mood, reduce stress and foster a sense of happiness and positivity. Just try laughing now, as an experiment. And keep laughing. Even if there was nothing originally funny to trigger the laughter, the endorphins will dutifully leap into action and in a matter of seconds you'll feel a surge of wellbeing. The same thing will happen with exercise.

Dopamine plays a key role in the brain's reward circuits. When released, it generates feelings of pleasure, satisfaction and excitement. The combination of these two neurotransmitters, both triggered by exercise, can significantly boost mood and motivation.

Exercise also increases blood flow to the brain, which raises levels of a protein called brain-derived neurotrophic factor (BDNF). This supports the production and maintenance of brain cells, contributing to improved mental clarity and cognitive function.

Insomnia & fatigue

While insomnia can often lead to fatigue, exercise will improve the quality of your sleep, by helping to regulate your circadian rhythm. If you sleep well, you'll feel more energized the next day. If you've had a bad night, you may not feel inclined to exercise. However, this would be a mistake: a recent study from the University of Portsmouth noted that 20 minutes of moderate exercise after a broken night will actually boost your brain power and improve cognitive function, so that you can effectively complete the tasks that await you.

How does exercise impact my menopause?

Exercise supports a healthy menopause in more ways than you might expect. There's a wealth of research highlighting how regular physical activity can alleviate symptoms and enhance both short- and long-term health and wellbeing. Introducing consistent exercise into your routine can transform the way you experience menopause.

- **Hot flushes:** Consistent exercise helps to reduce symptoms of hot flushes and night sweats, because of the role it plays in supporting a regular body temperature.
- **Mood management:** As we have seen above, the endorphins released by regular exercise help us to feel better, which will be a great help if hormonal fluctuations are affecting your mood and motivation.
- **Mental clarity:** By enhancing the supply of oxygen to the brain, exercise can play an important role in reducing symptoms of brain fog and poor memory.
- **Bone & muscle health:** Weight-bearing exercise and impact work, such as strength training, running or racquet sports, will all help to support optimal bone density. Reduced oestrogen levels during and post-menopause increase the risk of bone loss, which can lead to fractures. Resistance work and strength training will also help to support muscle mass, which can also start to decline during this phase of life.
- **Cardiovascular health:** The risk of cardiovascular disease increases post-menopause. A focus on regular aerobic exercise that activates the heart muscle, such as brisk walking, running, dancing, fast swimming or cycling, can all help to support heart health.
- **Weight management:** Along with a balanced diet, regular exercise will support weight management, which can often become a challenge as the metabolism slows down during the menopause.

HOW MUCH EXERCISE SHOULD I DO?

As we have seen above, two and a half hours of vigorous exercise each week is recommended. Any form of regular physical activity will support our energy levels, but when it comes to midlife and menopause, it's best to mix it up, because the requirements of our body are so broad. We need strength training and resistance work to support the loss of muscle tone and bone density during and post-menopause. We need cardiovascular work to support our heart health. We also need exercise that enhances flexibility, balance and core strength.

There is a tendency to stick with the form of exercise we're used to and feel competent at. Runners run. Swimmers swim. Lifters lift. Yogis do yoga. There often isn't a lot of crossover, and we can easily put ourselves in a box and stay within our comfort zone: "I'm not bendy", "I don't like the gym", "I can't run".

Here are some helpful activities to start scheduling into your daily or weekly routine.

Walking

A short brisk walk every day can make a world of difference, and you'll experience the benefits quite quickly, especially if you're not in the habit of exercising regularly. Aim for 20 minutes brisk walking at a rate of around 100 steps per minute. Set a timer on your phone and count the steps, so you can get a feel for the pace, and then head off! This will increase your heart rate and send that oxygen flooding around the body to promote energy production in your cells. It's something that you should be able to fit in easily during a lunch break or on your way to work, and it's a great habit to get into. Of course, if you're inclined to walk for longer, that's an added bonus, but make sure that you factor in 20 brisk minutes as part of that.

Cardiovascular activity

This could be running, fast swimming, tennis, dancing or anything else that gets your heart pumping. Choose something that you like, so that you're motivated to keep doing it. Cardiovascular activity will stimulate your mitochondria and enhance the energy production process. It will also promote a healthy blood pressure. High blood pressure affects the circulation of oxygen around the body. Left untreated, it will make the heart work harder and, while you might not notice the effect immediately, over time this will contribute to fatigue.

Strength training

Working with weights increases your muscle capacity and improves your strength and endurance, which means that you'll find daily activities less tiring. It will also help the flow of blood to the muscles, burning fat and supporting sustained energy levels. If you feel a little intimidated by the gym, you could try working with a personal trainer to get you started.

Yoga

Depending on the nature of the class, yoga may incorporate both cardiovascular and strength work, which would be a bonus. However, it's the breath work that is particularly interesting with yoga. The focus on deep, controlled breathing as you carry out each movement optimizes oxygen intake and helps to slow down a busy mind. This will improve mental clarity and focus. It also reduces levels of the stress hormone cortisol, which acts as an energy drain.

Free exercise

If you go to the gym faithfully three times per week but spend the rest of the time chained to your desk or sitting on the sofa, this will not help your cause. The standard recommended amount of vigorous exercise each week should be on top of, and not instead of, a generally active lifestyle. The recommended 10,000 steps every day is generally agreed to be an arbitrary figure, but it's not a bad indication of how much you're moving throughout the day. If you make a point of grasping opportunities for free exercise, this will provide regular stimulation for the mitochondria over the course of the day, which will help to keep your energy levels on track. Take the stairs instead of the elevator; walk up escalators; park further away from the supermarket; go over to speak to colleagues in the office instead of emailing them; use public transport instead of driving.

There are lots of ways you can embrace small opportunities for movement and the more you do that, the more your body will adapt to wanting to move.

Easy ways to increase your exercise

- **Audit your exercise output:** Be honest with yourself and calculate how much you're actually doing, rather than what you think you're doing. Then you can make a realistic plan.
- **Start small and take it step by step:** It may help to get some support from a personal trainer if you don't know where to start.
- **Get up an hour earlier** (this is easier during the summer months!) and go for an hour's walk in the park. It will stimulate your brain and activate your body so that you have a more productive day.

- **Get an exercise buddy:** It can be more motivating and more fun to team up with a friend to do your chosen activity.
- **If the gym isn't for you,** check out some of the excellent online exercise offerings that you can do in the privacy of your own home, such as Yoga With Adriene, Cara Fitness and Sam Palmer YouTube channels (see Resources, page 291). Start with bite-size options, such as a regular 15-minute session, to ease you into it.
- **Think outside the box:** If standard exercise options bore you, try something a bit different. Sign up to a dance class (even ballroom dancing can be surprisingly energetic); rediscover your inner child and order a skipping rope or a hula hoop; borrow a friend's dog and go for a long walk; or take up an active hobby, such as gardening.
- **If you function best with a target,** start with the classic 10,000 steps a day. You can use a free tracker app on your phone to keep count. Or sign up for a challenge, such as "walk a mile a day in January" to raise money for a charity.
- **Check out the Couch to 5K app:** You might surprise yourself. This app will take you on a gentle journey to being able to run 5k completely at your own pace. I'd never run in my life and honestly never thought I would, but during lockdown, at the age of 54, I tried it out. Now I really enjoy my very slow trot around the park, and I'm delighted by the benefits I feel.
- **A gym membership might suit you,** because it can be a one-stop shop for the range of recommended exercise types. Try shopping around, as there are some low-price options that can be very good value.
- **Don't sit at your desk for more than an hour:** Set a timer to remind you to get up and move around. This will improve circulation and stop you feeling tired and lethargic.

- **If urinary stress incontinence (leaking) is limiting your ability or motivation to exercise,** ask your doctor for a referral to a pelvic health physiotherapist who can help you manage and often resolve the issue. You can also use the Squeezy app for guidance on pelvic floor exercises (see Resources, page 291). This is a common problem that can be easily addressed, and it shouldn't stop you from staying active!

Energy Action Plan – my next steps

Do you need to move more? What are the realistic steps you could take to exercise more regularly to support your energy levels? Where could you start and how would you ensure that you stick to it?

Make a note of whatever stood out to you in this section and create a commitment to physical activity.

Focus on these three questions to create your SMART objectives:

1. What will I do?
2. How will I do it?
3. When will I do it by?

STRESS

Energy gain or energy drain? A little of one and an awful lot of the other is the reality of stress. There's no doubt that a small dose of stress, along with its associated hormones adrenaline and cortisol, can provide a temporary energy boost. It's often said that feeling a touch of nerves before a presentation or performance is beneficial, because it sharpens your focus and can lead to better results.

The stress response originated as a primitive reaction to physical danger, designed to help us survive imminent threats. It triggers an alarm within the body, releasing cortisol and adrenaline, which activate the fight-or-flight response. Heart rate increases, blood rushes to the muscles and a surge of energy or physical strength readies the body to tackle the perceived danger.

Once the threat passes, the stress hormones recede and the body returns to its normal state. But in modern life, true physical danger is rare. Instead, the stress response is often triggered by everyday challenges, such as a cancelled train, running late for an appointment or seeing your child's school pop up as an incoming call.

These daily challenges can lead to chronic stress, where cortisol levels remain consistently high. This persistent state rapidly depletes energy reserves, leaving you in a cycle of ongoing fatigue. Elevated cortisol disrupts the balance of the nervous system, keeping the sympathetic nervous system (responsible for "red alert") in overdrive. Meanwhile, the parasympathetic nervous system, which promotes calm and relaxation, takes a back seat.

Excessive stress impacts every system in the body by diverting resources away from what it deems non-essential. Blood flow is redirected to the muscles to help you run faster or fight more effectively, but this response often comes with a host of unexpected symptoms.

Over time, the prolonged activation of this stress response can lead to lasting damage, disrupting hormonal balance, affecting digestion, weakening the immune system and increasing the risk of chronic conditions such as cardiovascular disease and burnout.

Common signs of too much stress

- Insomnia
- Increased irritability
- Reduced tolerance for frustration
- Over-reaction to small issues
- Poor concentration and memory
- Loss of motivation
- Fatigue
- Difficulty switching off
- Loss of libido
- Digestive problems
- Recurring colds or infections
- High blood pressure
- Palpitations
- Headaches
- Abdominal weight gain
- Cravings for sugar or salt
- Teeth grinding or clenching
- Feeling overwhelmed or helpless

How does stress impact my energy levels?

Cortisol plays a crucial role in regulating our circadian rhythms and energy levels throughout the day. It is designed to start rising early in the morning, before we wake, to provide the energy needed for the day ahead. Over the course of the day, cortisol levels gradually decline, with a sharp drop around 10pm, preparing the body for sleep. Cortisol works in opposition to melatonin, the sleep–wake cycle hormone, which rises in the evening to promote drowsiness and declines in the morning to help us wake up.

When we are chronically stressed, cortisol levels remain elevated throughout the day and into the evening, making it difficult to switch off and rest. In severe cases, cortisol levels can become disrupted, leading to low levels in the morning – causing tiredness early in the day – and higher levels in the evening, which can leave you feeling more energetic when you should be winding down. This disrupts melatonin's action and interferes with the sleep–wake cycle.

High cortisol can also indirectly drain energy by interfering with the following systems and functions in the body:

- **Sleep:** As well as potentially delaying the onset of sleep, high cortisol can lead to night-time restlessness and fragmented sleep, resulting in wakefulness. It affects the quality of slow-wave sleep, the deep slumber required for physical repair and recovery. Elevated cortisol may lead to vivid or disturbing dreams, which will disrupt our sleep. It can also prolong the REM phase of sleep, which will affect our ability to lay down and consolidate new memories, impairing our cognitive function. All of this will leave you feeling tired, jaded and unproductive the following morning.

- **Digestion:** Stress has a direct impact on digestion, as blood is diverted away from the digestive tract during the fight-or-flight response. This slows down the action of the gut and affects nutrient absorption. If you're not absorbing the key nutrients that are required to support energy production, this will have a significant impact on your vitality. Stress is also a common trigger for IBS symptoms, such as bloating, which can leave you feeling pretty lethargic.
- **Metabolism:** Excessive levels of cortisol keep the body in a constant state of alert, ready for action at any moment. To maintain a readily available supply of energy for the fight-or-flight response, the body prioritizes storing food as abdominal fat rather than converting it into energy for everyday use. So too much stress will lead to a combination of fatigue and weight gain.

How does stress impact my menopause?

Stress really is the enemy during menopause. The more stressed you are, the worse your symptoms are likely to be. It's a simple equation. This is a time in life when prioritizing self-care and stress management becomes more important than ever.

The reason lies in how stress directly affects the body's "Plan B" as we transition through perimenopause and menopause. I dedicate an entire chapter to managing this issue in my book *The Happy Menopause: Smart Nutrition to Help You Flourish.*

In short, the body has back-up systems for nearly everything. It is programmed to maintain balance through the process of homeostasis, the delicate regulation of fluid levels, temperature, blood sugar, blood pressure, calcium levels and more.

Homeostasis also governs hormone balance. As oestrogen production in the ovaries declines, the adrenal glands step in, producing a weak form of oestrogen designed to support us through mid- and later life.

So far, so good. But the adrenal glands are also responsible for the stress response, releasing cortisol and adrenaline as needed. This process always takes precedence, as the fight-or-flight response is essential for survival.

If you're chronically stressed, your adrenal glands become preoccupied with producing cortisol and adrenaline. This leaves little capacity for producing the oestrogen your body needs, exacerbating menopausal symptoms.

Chronic stress & the mitochondria

Prolonged exposure to stress can have profound effects on mitochondrial function. It often results in oxidative damage to mitochondrial DNA, which disrupts the mitochondria's ability to produce the ATP molecules that power our energy levels. This not only reduces energy production but also hampers overall cellular efficiency, which will create further fatigue. Chronic stress also impairs the regeneration of mitochondria, slowing down the processes vital for maintaining energy and cellular health.

DIETARY STRATEGIES TO MANAGE STRESS

There are several ways your diet can help regulate stress levels, but this works best as part of a broader programme targeting the root causes of your stress. Diet alone can't remove stress, but the right foods can build resilience, helping you feel better equipped to handle the challenges of your daily life.

Here are some key areas to focus on to support your nervous system and regulate your body's response to stress:

Blood sugar balance

For me, this is Nutrition 101 when it comes to stress management. Every time your blood sugar crashes, your body releases cortisol and adrenaline. If you're already dealing with stress, those extra stress hormones won't help! Maintaining stable blood sugar levels will help keep them in check. (See page 113 for more information on balancing blood sugar.)

Adrenal support

Your adrenal glands burn through B vitamins and vitamin C when you're stressed. Eating foods rich in these key nutrients helps ensure your adrenal glands function effectively without going into overdrive. This supports the production of cortisol and adrenaline in a balanced way.

The minimum daily requirement for vitamin C is 40mg, just enough to prevent scurvy! However, most people require significantly more for optimal health, particularly during periods of stress or illness. The best sources of vitamin C are vegetables, with raw red peppers providing approximately 190mg per 100g – nearly three times the amount found in an orange (53mg per 100g). Dark green leafy vegetables, such as kale, are also excellent sources, offering around 120mg per 100g. While oranges are a good source, other fruits such as kiwi (92mg per 100g) and strawberries (59mg per 100g) are also rich in vitamin C. Parsley is also an excellent source, providing 130mg per 100g. You can find out more about sources of B vitamins on page 168.

Magnesium

This is nature's calmer. It supports your nervous system and acts as a buffer against the stresses of daily life. Optimal magnesium levels can enhance your resilience, regulate stress and even help with sleep issues. If you struggle to switch off at night, magnesium may be your best friend. (Learn more about this marvellous mineral on page 171.)

L-theanine

This compound found in tea has a naturally calming effect on the body. It promotes relaxation without causing drowsiness, making it an excellent addition to your stress-management toolkit. When combined with caffeine, which is also present in tea, L-theanine helps balance the stimulating effects, reducing the jitters or anxiety that caffeine can sometimes cause.

Omega-3 fatty acids

Found in oily fish, flaxseeds and walnuts, omega-3s support brain health and help reduce stress by playing a crucial role in the functioning of the nervous system (see page 53 for more on essential fatty acids).

Hydration

Dehydration can amplify feelings of stress and fatigue. Ensure you're drinking enough water throughout the day to support overall wellbeing (see pages 78–9).

Caffeine

A powerful stimulant, excessive caffeine can overstimulate your nervous system, increase your heart rate and trigger the unnecessary release of stress hormones. Limiting your intake (see page 218) is a simple way to support your body during stressful times.

Alcohol

Excessive alcohol consumption adds stress to the body, both physically and mentally. Reducing your intake (see page 229) can help lighten the load on your system and improve your overall resilience.

Avoid fasting

Intermittent fasting is a popular strategy for weight management. While this can be effective for some individuals, fasting is not recommended for anyone who is chronically stressed. The perceived state of starvation can raise cortisol levels, putting further strain on the adrenal glands.

LIFESTYLE STRATEGIES FOR MANAGING STRESS

Human beings are highly adaptable, which often means we adjust to – and put up with – situations or issues that, with some distance, we would recognize as simply unacceptable.

If you suspect stress is contributing to your fatigue, it's helpful to take some time to reflect on what may be adding to your mental load. In my nutrition clinic, I often meet women who either don't recognize they're stressed or claim to thrive on it, when this is often visibly not the case.

While it's not always practical or possible to remove specific causes of stress, if changes are possible, that should be a sensible first step. However, you can still make a significant difference by focusing on the areas of your life you *can* influence.

Take control of your diary

Are you a "yes" person? If so, it's time to become a bit more ruthless about managing your schedule.

- **Scheduling back-to-back meetings:** This is not a smart move. Allowing yourself time to breathe or take a short comfort break between meetings can ease the sense of overwhelm.
- **Blocking out time:** Get out your diary or family calendar and block out one entire weekend each month when you're not committing to anything at all in advance. You can use this time for self-care, quality family time or a spontaneous treat. Knowing that you have a regular haven of nothingness awaiting you will help you feel more grounded.
- **Dare to say no:** Practise saying no if needed, preparing a phrase that you can confidently use if you're accustomed to accommodating others. Overloading yourself impacts your adrenal glands, and simplifying your commitments will benefit your overall wellbeing.

Choose relaxing activities

"What do you do to relax?" is a question I ask every woman who visits my nutrition clinic. It's astonishing how often I'm met with an awkward silence and a slight look of panic when they realize they're not at all sure how to answer.

- **Calm & distraction:** Think of an activity that takes you out of yourself – something that brings you joy. Whether it's painting, crafting, ballroom dancing, playing a musical instrument or baking, finding something that fully absorbs you and engages a different part of your brain can provide relief from worries. Once you find what works for you, make it a regular part of your schedule.

- **Complementary therapies:** Let someone else take the load off. Therapies such as reflexology, acupuncture, hypnotherapy and aromatherapy are known for their supportive role in stress reduction. Even a simple massage can be incredibly relaxing. Consider a monthly treatment, as a little self-care goes a long way.

- **Yoga, mindfulness & meditation:** Breathwork in yoga sequences helps focus the mind and can be a great aid in calming an overactive nervous system. Try paced breathing – slowing down your breaths to about 7 breaths per minute instead of the usual 13–14. This can be done discreetly at your desk or on public transport when feeling stressed or anxious. Studies show simple paced breathing can significantly reduce stress levels. You might also explore mindfulness or meditation apps, which offer extensive research-backed benefits for mood and mental health.

- **Walking in nature:** Even a short walk in a natural setting, particularly among trees, can help lower cortisol levels. This is a simple beneficial addition to your daily life that you can easily incorporate without disrupting your schedule.

- **Exercise:** This is a double-edged sword when it comes to stress. Regular, moderate exercise helps reduce cortisol and supports stress management. However, intense exercise such as high-intensity interval training (HIIT) or spin classes can actually raise cortisol levels and put additional strain on the adrenal glands. Extreme workouts are best avoided if you are chronically stressed, particularly in the evening, when cortisol levels should start reducing.

- **Sleep:** Prioritizing good-quality sleep is essential for managing stress. There's a direct correlation between poor sleep and increased cortisol levels. In the next section, we'll explore the role of sleep in more detail.

Easy ways to lower stress levels

- **Have an Epsom salts bath or footbath:** Epsom salts are magnesium sulphate. Add 2–3 handfuls to a bath or footbath and soak for about 20 minutes. The magnesium is absorbed through the skin, helping restore your equilibrium after a stressful day and setting you up for a good night's sleep.
- **Add a twice-daily breathwork reminder to your phone:** Take a moment to do a paced breathing exercise at your desk.
- **Download a mindfulness or meditation app:** Try out the 1-minute or 5-minute options to get started. Two popular options are Calm and Headspace.
- **Take a red pen to your diary NOW:** Start blocking out time for yourself, whether it's an evening, a weekend or just 30 minutes each day.
- **Book a recurring appointment with your favourite complementary therapist:** Prioritize self-care with regular sessions.
- **Think about what brings you joy:** Take time to identify activities that make you happy and find small ways to incorporate more of them into your routine.
- **Re-read the section on blood sugar balance (page 113):** Create a stress-busting meal plan for yourself to keep your energy stable and avoid additional strain on your body.
- **Enlist the help of family and friends:** Let them know you're taking steps to manage stress – if you tell them, it's likely that they'll be more supportive of the changes you're making.
- **Speak to your employer if work is causing stress:** Reach out to your line manager, HR team or occupational health department. There may be more support available than you realize.
- **Step outside for fresh air and a walk:** A brisk walk, especially in a natural setting, can clear your mind and lower cortisol levels.
- **Spend time with people who make you laugh:** A good belly laugh is proven to reduce cortisol levels.

- **Try journaling before bed:** Write down your worries or to-do list to clear your mind and make it easier to relax.
- **Practise gratitude:** Spend a minute or two each day reflecting on three things you're grateful for – it can shift your mindset and lower stress.
- **Declutter your surroundings:** A tidy space can help reduce feelings of overwhelm and create a calming environment.
- **Play uplifting music or listen to a podcast:** This can act as a positive distraction and elevate your mood.

Energy Action Plan – my next steps

It's important to start slowly and avoid being overly ambitious. If you're already feeling stressed, the last thing you need to do is to add to your sense of overwhelm. Take some time to reflect on the main sources of your stress and choose two or three actions from the list above that feel most relevant to your situation.

Make a note of whatever stood out to you in this section and create a commitment to self-care.

Focus on these three questions to create your SMART objectives:

1. What will I do?
2. How will I do it?
3. When will I do it by?

SLEEP

How well do you sleep? Prioritizing your sleep really is a no-brainer when it comes to looking for an energy gain. We all know that a good night's sleep will leave us feeling energized, positive, sharp and productive, whereas a bad night's sleep will do quite the opposite. If you're consistently feeling tired, it's important to consider whether a lack of sleep, or poor-quality sleep, is a part of the picture.

Sleep is fundamental to our health and wellbeing, and its influence stretches far beyond simply providing us with the rest that we need, although that is very important, of course.

While we sleep, the body is hard at work undertaking a whole range of restorative processes that influence brain health, consolidate memory, support the immune system, promote healing and recovery of tissues and muscles, and play a key role in weight management.

If we miss out on our sleep, the long-term consequences will stretch far beyond a lack of energy.

Sleep cycles

Our sleep consists of a series of 90-minute cycles over the course of the night. Each stage of the cycle will include a sequence of reactions and activities that support our overall health, which is why a complete cycle is so important. When you wake up during the night, the current sleep cycle is disrupted and will start again once you fall asleep. Persistent wakefulness will cause a series of broken cycles, leaving you feeling unrefreshed in the morning.

The sleep cycle broadly breaks down into two parts: non-rapid eye movement (REM) sleep and REM sleep. Non-REM sleep has three phases:

- **Light sleep:** This is a transitional phase which only lasts a few moments. It gets the body ready for deeper sleep and initiates the repair and recovery process.
- **Deeper light sleep:** In this phase the heart rate slows, the body temperature drops and the metabolic rate decreases, to conserve energy. The brain prepares for the process of memory consolidation, in which it lays down the memories we have acquired during the day. This phase lasts for roughly 45 minutes.
- **Deep sleep or slow-wave sleep:** This is the most restorative phase of the cycle and is essential for feeling refreshed. Repair and recovery processes take place and the immune system is reinforced. The brain undertakes a self-cleaning process, removing waste products that have built up over the course of the day, and which may contribute to chronic conditions such as dementia or Alzheimer's disease.

REM sleep follows deep sleep, before the cycle completes and the body goes on to start a new one. It is during this phase that we might have vivid dreams. REM sleep is important for memory consolidation and for making neural connections that support creativity and enhance problem solving.

As the night progresses, the length of REM sleep varies: it tends to be shorter in the early part of the night, as the body prioritizes deep sleep, and becomes longer as morning approaches, to prepare for waking. REM sleep represents around 20–25 per cent of our overall sleep.

The cumulative benefits of completing multiple sleep cycles also include blood sugar balance and the regulation of hormones that govern appetite, supporting weight management; emotional resilience and a reduced risk of mental health issues; a healthy blood pressure; and reduced inflammation.

Typical signs of insufficient sleep

- Tiredness
- Feeling unrefreshed in the morning
- Irritability
- Low mood or depression
- Anxiety
- Poor concentration and memory
- A tendency to make mistakes
- Lack of creativity

- Frequent colds or infections
- Poor wound healing
- Weight gain
- Cravings for sugar or carbohydrate
- Increased appetite
- Poor balance or lack of coordination
- Loss of strength and stamina
- Increased sensitivity to pain

How does lack of sleep affect my energy levels?

You can see from the explanation above that sleep plays multiple roles in supporting both our physical and mental energy.

If we don't get enough sleep, it directly impacts our physical energy levels by reducing strength, impairing coordination and affecting endurance. This can make us more prone to minor accidents, such as slipping, tripping or falling, as well as slow down physical recovery from exercise or injuries. In the long term, chronic sleep deprivation may increase the risk of health issues such as cardiovascular disease, weakened immunity and weight gain, which will indirectly affect our energy levels.

Sleep is equally crucial for our mental energy. Without sufficient rest, brain function becomes impaired, leading to poor memory, loss of focus and a reduced ability to think creatively or solve problems. Decision-making suffers, emotional regulation becomes harder and we may feel more irritable, impatient or stressed. Over time, persistent sleep deprivation can significantly increase the risk of anxiety, depression and other mental health issues.

Ultimately, quality sleep is the foundation for physical vitality and mental sharpness, and without it, every aspect of our daily performance is affected.

Sleep & the mitochondria

Sleep is essential for maintaining healthy mitochondrial function. During the restorative phases of sleep, mitochondria undergo repair and renewal, ensuring efficient ATP production. Sleep also reduces oxidative stress and supports the removal of damaged mitochondria through a process called mitophagy, protecting cells from dysfunction. In contrast, poor sleep disrupts these critical processes, leading to impaired energy production, increased oxidative damage and a heightened risk of chronic conditions associated with mitochondrial dysfunction.

Menopause & sleep: a two-way struggle

Our menopause and our sleep are intricately linked, with each influencing the other in significant ways. You can see below the different ways in which the menopause affects our sleep, and how lack of sleep, in turn, may exacerbate menopausal symptoms:

How menopause affects the quality of our sleep

- **Hot flushes and night sweats,** triggered by the declining levels of oestrogen, are a very common sleep disruptor during the perimenopause. For some women these issues may persist post-menopause.
- **Hormonal surges** during the night can commonly trigger wakefulness, even without a hot flush.
- **Fluctuating levels of progesterone** can make it harder to fall asleep and stay asleep. They may also contribute to feelings of anxiety which may lead to insomnia.
- **Changes in the bladder,** or issues with urinary stress incontinence (leaking) due to a weakened pelvic floor muscle, may increase urinary frequency, interrupting sleep for a visit to the bathroom.
- **A change of circadian rhythm** during menopause may affect the body clock and disrupts the sleep–wake cycle.

How poor sleep affects our menopause symptoms

- While hot flushes can cause wakefulness, the reverse is also true, creating a vicious cycle of insomnia. Sleep deprivation can increase instances of hot flushes and night sweats during perimenopause.
- Impaired cognitive function: Issues with brain fog and poor concentration are common symptoms for some women during menopause, and these symptoms will be aggravated by lack of sleep.
- Insomnia will reduce mental resilience and emotional wellbeing, contributing to symptoms of anxiety, low mood or mood swings.
- The lower pain thresholds caused by chronic lack of sleep can make menopausal joint and muscle pain much more uncomfortable.
- Changes in metabolism and weight gain are common concerns for women in midlife, and insomnia can make this even more challenging. Poor sleep disrupts the appetite-regulating hormones leptin and ghrelin, which can lead to an increased appetite.

Potential causes of poor sleep

- Going to bed too late and getting up too early
- Struggling to switch off and fall asleep
- Stress and anxiety
- Hormonal surges and hot flushes or sweats
- A noisy environment
- Too much light in the bedroom
- The bedroom being too hot or too cold
- Eating a heavy meal late at night
- Alcohol and caffeine – known sleep disruptors
- Using digital devices in the bedroom
- Perimenopause

DIETARY STRATEGIES TO SUPPORT SLEEP

What and when we eat and drink can significantly affect the quality of our sleep. Just a few simple changes could make a world of difference to your slumber. These are some of the key areas to consider, to ensure that your diet is as conducive as possible to a good night's sleep.

Blood sugar balance

If you have no problem dropping off to sleep, but regularly wake up at around 2–3am for no obvious reason, there's a good chance that it's related to low blood sugar. Tucking into sugary treats and processed foods in the evening, or having a meal that contains little or no protein and large portions of refined carbohydrate, such as white rice or white pasta, may lead to a spike in blood sugar by bedtime.

This will trigger a hormonal response which ultimately results in the release of cortisol, a hormone that induces wakefulness at the very time when you should be deeply asleep. Addressing the balance of your meals and snacks in the evening can resolve this problem relatively quickly. Check back to the detailed advice on page 118 about the foods to focus on and the foods to avoid in order to maintain blood sugar balance.

Timing

It's important not to go to bed either hungry or overfull. In either case, this will lead to wakefulness. If you tend to eat very early in the evening, you might benefit from a small snack before bed, such as a banana with 4 or 5 nuts, if you're prone to insomnia. Avoiding eating heavy or rich foods in the evening will help to sidestep issues of indigestion or bloating that could hinder your sleep. Stay hydrated throughout the day, because dehydration can disrupt sleep. However, avoiding drinking large amounts of fluid close to bedtime will help to reduce the risk of night-time bathroom trips.

SLEEP-FRIENDLY FOODS	
What?	**Why?**
Wholegrains, e.g. brown rice, wholewheat pasta, sweet potato, vegetables AND Meat, fish, eggs, tofu, pulses, nuts or seeds	These complex carbohydrates provide sustained energy for the body, which promotes blood sugar balance. Combining complex carbohydrates with protein at the evening meal will support blood sugar balance.

SLEEP-FRIENDLY FOODS

What?	Why?
Spinach, Swiss chard, rocket/arugula, almonds, sunflower seeds, wholegrains	These foods are rich in magnesium which will be helpful for anyone who struggles to switch off and fall asleep. Magnesium helps to support the nervous system, promote relaxation and calm the mind, readying the body for sleep.
Chicken, turkey, oats, banana, dairy products, nuts	These are good sources of tryptophan, the amino acid required for the production of melatonin, which regulates our sleep–wake cycle.
Cherries, pistachios, walnuts, eggs, fish	These foods promote melatonin levels in the body, the hormone that governs the sleep–wake cycle.

SLEEP-FRIENDLY DRINKS

What?	Why?
Camomile tea	This contains an antioxidant called apigenin, which helps to promote relaxation and sleep.
Warm milk	A traditional remedy which can work well, due to the high levels of tryptophan in milk.
Tart cherry juice	Extracted from the Montmorency cherry, this supports melatonin production. It's commonly found in health-food stores.

SLEEP-FRIENDLY DRINKS	
What?	**Why?**
Herbal teas, such as valerian, lavender, passionflower and lemon balm	These all have calming properties and can help to quieten a busy mind and prepare the body for sleep.
Decaffeinated green tea	This is a good source of L-theanine, a compound that can be very helpful in calming the nervous system and readying the body for sleep.

Foods and habits to avoid to support your sleep

- Caffeine is a powerful stimulant and known sleep disruptor (see page 212). Avoiding caffeinated drinks, such as coffee, tea, cola or energy drinks in the evening, will reduce the risk of sleep disturbances.
- Alcohol may initially have a sedative effect; however, it disrupts sleep cycles over the course of the night, affecting the quality of your slumber. It takes about an hour to metabolize each unit of alcohol, and once this process is complete, wakefulness can follow.
- Sugary and processed foods, which will lead to a blood sugar spike and crash, can cause you to wake up in the night.
- Spicy, acidic or rich foods may cause indigestion or heartburn, which will interfere with sleep.
- Aged cheeses, cured meats and fermented foods, such as kimchi or sauerkraut, are best avoided in the evening, if you find it hard to sleep. These contain the amino acid tyramine, which stimulates the release of noradrenaline, which increases the heart rate and can create a state of alertness that is not compatible with sleep.

LIFESTYLE STRATEGIES TO SUPPORT SLEEP

Making a few simple changes to your bedtime routine and night-time environment can really help to improve the quality of your sleep. Here are some suggestions:

Optimize your sleep environment

Is your bedroom a sleep-friendly zone? Take a good look at it – is it a relaxing haven or does it double up as a workspace? What could you do to ensure that your body instinctively sees it as a place of rest? Opt for blackout blinds or curtains so there's no light disturbance, or consider using an eye mask. If noise is an issue, you may benefit from ear plugs.

Does your bedding need an overhaul? If you regularly experience hot flushes and sweats, then it may be more effective to have layers of bedding, rather than one thick quilt.

Ban digital devices from the bedroom. It's possible that the blue light may interfere with the action of melatonin, the drowsiness-promoting hormone. What's more, when I chatted to Russell Foster, Professor of Circadian Neuroscience for The Happy Menopause podcast, he explained that the stimulation provided by your phone was an even bigger issue. Checking your phone, even just to see the time, if you wake in the night will automatically stimulate the brain and make it harder to get back to sleep. Perhaps it's time for an old-fashioned alarm clock instead.

Create a sleep routine

Prepare yourself for bed in the same way that you would a small child. Our inner five-year-old still requires that wind-down time. Put away digital devices at least an hour before bed, so that your brain is not in overdrive. Opt for relaxing activities, such as reading, listening to soft music, taking a warm bath or watching TV, but nothing too hectic or disturbing.

Gentle exercise, such as a short walk or some yoga stretches, can help to promote relaxation, but avoid intense exercise later in the evening, because this will increase cortisol levels and lead to a state of overstimulation.

Turn the lights down: the last room we visit before bed is usually the bathroom, which often has glaringly bright lighting. Bright light can trick your body into thinking it's daytime and may disrupt melatonin signalling just when you need it most.

Try going to bed and getting up at the same time each day. Studies have shown that this regular approach can help to programme the body to be ready for sleep.

Go outside in the morning as early as possible after getting up. The exposure to morning light on the eyes helps to regulate the circadian rhythms and the sleep–wake cycle. This is particularly effective for anyone suffering from jetlag.

Experiment with complementary therapies

Aromatherapy and the use of essential oils may help to promote sleep. Try a few drops of lavender oil on your pillow or in a diffuser.

Therapies such as acupuncture, reflexology, massage therapy or hypnotherapy can be very effective for anyone who experiences chronic insomnia. A restorative yoga or tai chi practice can also be very calming.

Look into mindfulness, meditation or breathing exercises that you could practise during the day and then apply easily if you wake up in the night. There are lots of good options to choose from; the Headspace and Calm apps might be a helpful place to start.

Explore sound therapy: for example, by using a white noise machine, or playing sounds of nature, such as rainfall or ocean waves. You may want to download Max Richter's Sleep, an eight-hour lullaby composed in consultation with a neurologist, designed to support the subconscious mind and enhance sleep (see Resources, page 291).

Easy ways to improve your sleep

- Balance your blood sugar in the evening.
- Avoid caffeine after 11am.
- Eliminate alcohol altogether.
- Create a calming pre-bedtime routine.
- Avoid using digital devices for at least an hour before bed.
- Banish your phone from the bedroom.
- Make your bedroom a sleep-friendly environment.

Energy Action Plan – my next steps

You can see how many different factors can affect our sleep. Which ones stood out to you? Are there two or three key actions that you could start on straightaway? Sleep really is the cornerstone that supports our energy levels, so if you can get this right, it could make a big difference to your brain and your body.

Make a note of whatever stood out to you in this section and create a commitment to improving your sleep.

Focus on these three questions to create your SMART objectives:

1. What will I do?
2. How will I do it?
3. When will I do it by?

INFLAMMATION

Inflammation is the first line of defence of the immune system, acting as a protective mechanism to keep us fit and well. If we injure ourselves or pick up an infection, the immune system will activate our white blood cells and trigger them to release chemicals called cytokines, which promote tissue repair and fight off any harmful pathogens. These chemicals generate redness, swelling or heat around the site of injury.

This is designed to be a short-lived, beneficial response – an important part of the healing process before everything returns to normal. So far, so good.

However, inflammation doesn't always switch off as it should. In some cases, it may occur even without the trigger of an injury or infection. Chronic low-level activation of the immune system can cause physiological damage and niggling health issues; it can also lead to an autoimmune condition, where an overactive immune system may actually attack body tissues; and it is at the root of many chronic health conditions, such as cardiovascular disease and cancer. It is also increasingly linked to instances of chronic fatigue syndrome or ME.

Common signs of low-grade inflammation

- Persistent fatigue
- Joint pain
- Muscle aches
- Digestive issues
- Weight gain
- Headaches
- A sense of malaise
- Sinusitis
- Eczema, psoriasis or dermatitis
- Weight gain
- High blood pressure
- Allergies
- Brain fog
- Low mood

How does inflammation affect my energy levels?

As a normal part of the immune system's protective response, inflammation should not affect our energy levels on a day-to-day basis. However, a state of chronic low-grade inflammation can be extremely draining on the body and lead to a persistent lack of energy.

Inflammation can often be at the root of a condition that doctors call TATT (Tired All The Time), when other more obvious potential causes of fatigue have been ruled out.

Any defence mechanism in the body will always take priority because it's the body's job to keep us alive. If the immune system stays on high alert, this diverts energy stores away from everyday functions and activities to power the protective response. This will leave you feeling tired and unproductive.

Chronic inflammation will also place the body under undue stress, disrupting the balance of cortisol. Additionally, the blood sugar mechanism can be affected, impairing the insulin response and reducing our ability to draw energy from the food we eat. It's also very common to experience brain fog and mental fatigue in a state of persistent inflammation.

Inflammation & the mitochondria

The persistent release of cytokines caused by chronic inflammation can disrupt mitochondrial function, affecting energy production at a cellular level. Increased levels of oxidative stress can also damage mitochondria and hinder the generation of new ones.

What causes inflammation?

- **Dietary factors:** Processed foods, junk food, trans fats, excessive sugar and alcohol are all pro-inflammatory. High levels of grains, red meat, dairy and saturated fats in the diet may also stimulate inflammation.
- **Chronic Stress:** This increases the production of inflammatory cytokines.
- **Excess weight:** Abdominal fat increases inflammatory markers in the body.
- **Chronic or unresolved infections:** These include issues such as gum disease, bacterial infections in the gut or persistent viral infections.
- **A food sensitivity:** An unidentified food intolerance or allergy will trigger an inflammatory response.
- **Lack of physical activity:** A sedentary lifestyle increases inflammatory markers in the body.
- **Lifestyle factors:** Insomnia, dehydration, nicotine, excessive alcohol and caffeine can all increase levels of inflammation.
- **Environmental factors:** Exposure to pollutants and chemicals can promote inflammation.

How does the menopause affect inflammation?

Oestrogen has anti-inflammatory properties, and as levels gradually decline during perimenopause and menopause, the body becomes more susceptible to chronic inflammation. This can worsen common symptoms such as brain fog, fatigue and joint pain. Additionally, fat distribution changes during menopause, with an increase in abdominal fat – a metabolically active tissue that can trigger the release of inflammatory cytokines.

Hot flushes and night sweats can contribute to disturbed sleep, and persistent insomnia further exacerbates inflammation. The increased propensity for inflammation during this stage of life impacts energy levels and overall wellbeing, making it crucial to adopt an anti-inflammatory approach to both diet and lifestyle.

DIETARY STRATEGIES TO REDUCE INFLAMMATION

Limiting your exposure to pro-inflammatory foods and promoting an anti-inflammatory diet can help to reduce the inflammatory load on your body.

EXAMPLES OF PRO-INFLAMMATORY FOODS TO AVOID	
Food	**Impact**
Sugar and refined carbohydrates (e.g. white bread, baked goods)	These will cause a blood sugar spike, which can trigger the release of cytokines.

EXAMPLES OF PRO-INFLAMMATORY FOODS TO AVOID

Food	Impact
Processed food, junk food or fast food, e.g. crisps, deep-fried chicken, doughnuts, cookies	May contain trans fats, which are highly inflammatory.
Processed meats, e.g. sausages, bacon or salami	These contain high levels of saturated fats, which stimulate inflammation.
Grains that contain gluten, e.g. wheat, rye, barley	These can trigger an inflammatory response in people with coeliac disease or who have a sensitivity to gluten.
Full-fat dairy, e.g. cheese or cream	The high levels of saturated fats may trigger inflammation. Individuals who are sensitive to lactose or cow's milk protein may experience inflammation.
Nightshade vegetables, e.g. potatoes, peppers, tomatoes, aubergine/eggplant	These may trigger an inflammatory response and cause joint pain for anyone who is sensitive to nightshades.
Excessive alcohol	This creates oxidative stress, which will lead to inflammation.

EXAMPLES OF PRO-INFLAMMATORY FOODS TO AVOID

Food	Impact
Refined oils, such as corn or sunflower oil	These are high in omega-6 fatty acids, which can disrupt the omega-6:omega-3 ratio and increase inflammatory mediators.

EXAMPLES OF ANTI-INFLAMMATORY FOODS TO PRIORITIZE

Food	Impact
Omega-3 fatty acids, found in salmon, sardines, flaxseed and walnuts	These support anti-inflammatory pathways and promote the correct ratio of omega-6:omega-3.
Wholegrains, e.g. unprocessed oats, quinoa	High-fibre foods support a healthy gut microbiome and help to reduce inflammation.
Pulses, e.g. lentils, chickpeas/ garbanzo beans, beans	These lean proteins are rich in fibre and low in inflammatory saturated fats.
Green vegetables, e.g. spinach, kale, broccoli	Green vegetables are rich in antioxidants and polyphenols that help to combat inflammation.

EXAMPLES OF ANTI-INFLAMMATORY FOODS TO PRIORITIZE	
Food	**Impact**
Live natural yogurt	This a good source of beneficial bacteria that supports gut health and moderates inflammation.
Extra virgin olive oil	An excellent source of anti-inflammatory monounsaturates and antioxidants.
Turmeric	This contains curcumin, a powerful anti-inflammatory compound.
Raw, unsalted nuts, e.g. almonds, walnuts	These are an excellent source of anti-inflammatory omega-3 fatty acids. They also contain a number of antioxidants that help to combat inflammation.

The Mediterranean diet

The Mediterranean diet is an anti-inflammatory eating approach inspired by the cuisines of countries bordering the Mediterranean Sea, such as Greece, Italy and Spain. A large body of evidence highlights the benefits of this diet, including its role in lowering inflammatory markers, improving heart health and reducing the risk of chronic disease.

This diet can be particularly effective for women during perimenopause and menopause, a time when low-grade inflammation caused by the drop in oestrogen may affect overall health.

The diet focuses on wholefoods that are minimally processed, nutrient-rich and naturally anti-inflammatory. It emphasizes fresh vegetables, healthy fats from oily fish and olive oil, wholegrains, legumes, nuts and seeds. Moderate consumption of eggs, dairy and poultry is encouraged, while red and processed meats are limited.

Here are some examples of how you could include the Mediterranean approach in your daily meal plans.

Meal	Example 1	Example 2
Breakfast	Authentic Greek yogurt with berries and 1 tablespoon walnuts or ground flaxseed	Wholegrain toast with avocado, tomatoes and a poached egg
Lunch	Grilled salmon or sardine salad with watercress, rocket/arugula, olives and red onion, with an olive oil and lemon dressing	A wholegrain pitta bread, stuffed with falafel, tzatziki, lettuce and tomatoes
Dinner	Lentil or bean casserole, with spinach, tomato and garlic	Grilled chicken or crispy tofu with roasted vegetables and quinoa
Snacks	6–7 almonds with a clementine	Cucumber slices with houmous or tahini
Dessert	A small portion of ricotta cheese with honey and crushed pistachios	Sliced nectarine drizzled with a small amount of melted dark chocolate

Anti-inflammatory supplements

Supplements might seem like a quick fix for reducing inflammation, but they should be approached with caution. If you have any medical conditions or are taking medication, it's important to check with your doctor before starting any new supplements. Some common anti-inflammatory supplements can interfere with heart medications and other drugs.

Assuming you've been given the all-clear, here are some options that may help:

Omega-3

Choose a pure fish oil supplement (rather than fish liver oil, which may contain toxins). If you follow a plant-based diet, algae oil is an excellent alternative to ensure sufficient EPA and DHA, the key anti-inflammatory compounds in omega-3.

Turmeric

Rich in curcumin, a powerful anti-inflammatory compound, turmeric may be particularly effective in alleviating joint pain. For better absorption, choose a supplement that includes black pepper (piperine) or is labelled as formulated for bioavailability.

Vitamin D

Deficiency in vitamin D has been linked to higher levels of inflammatory markers. Supplementing this essential vitamin is especially important in regions with limited sunlight exposure.

Magnesium

This helps regulate the stress response, improve sleep quality and support overall muscle and nerve function, reducing inflammation indirectly.

Ginger

Known for its anti-inflammatory and antioxidant properties, ginger supplements or extracts may help with issues such as joint pain and digestive inflammation.

Probiotics

Supporting a healthy gut microbiome can help modulate inflammation throughout the body. Look for a multi-strain probiotic with a range of different bacteria, but beware of very high doses of over 50 billion bacteria. These may cause digestive discomfort in sensitive individuals. A lower dose taken consistently over two to three months is often more effective and more comfortable.

LIFESTYLE STRATEGIES FOR MANAGING INFLAMMATION

There are four key lifestyle pillars to help resolve issues of low-grade inflammation:

Physical activity

Regular moderate exercise lowers inflammation by reducing visceral fat and supporting healthy immune function. Daily walking, swimming or maintaining a regular yoga practice are all excellent options (see pages 238–40 for more ideas).

Stress management

Chronic stress disrupts immune function and aggravates the inflammatory response. Simple practices such as slow breathing, mindfulness or meditation can help reduce stress levels (see pages 248–52 for more advice).

Sleep hygiene

Chronic sleep deprivation can trigger an inflammatory response. To improve sleep quality, ensure your bedroom is a calm, sleep-friendly environment; maintain a consistent sleep schedule, even on weekends; and limit screen time and exposure to blue light before bed. (See pages 262–4 for more sleep tips.)

Support for gut health

A healthy balance of gut bacteria helps to modulate the immune function and reduce inflammation. Foods that are rich in probiotics, e.g. kefir or kimchi, or prebiotics, e.g. onions and garlic, can help to support a healthy digestive tract.

Easy ways to reduce inflammation

- Follow a Mediterranean diet.
- Audit your diet for pro-inflammatory foods and prepare an anti-inflammatory meal plan for the week.
- Schedule in regular moderate exercise.
- Prioritize stress management.
- Support your sleep with a sleep hygiene programme.
- Reduce your alcohol consumption.
- Show your gut some love by increasing fibre and probiotic foods in your diet.
- Consider a food intolerance test to rule out any potential trigger foods.

Energy Action Plan – my next steps

Do you think low-grade inflammation might be a factor in your lack of energy? It's actually a fairly common issue, especially for women in midlife. What stood out to you in this section? Are there some obvious quick wins you can achieve that could help to reduce your inflammatory markers? Pick two or three key actions. For example, is your diet markedly pro-inflammatory? Perhaps you'd benefit from following a Mediterranean diet.

Make a note of whatever stood out to you in this section and create a commitment to reducing inflammation.

Focus on these three questions to create your SMART objectives:

1. What will I do?
2. How will I do it?
3. When will I do it by?

From insight to action: get ready to design your Energy Action Plan

Throughout this chapter, you've seen the powerful ways your lifestyle choices can shape your physical and mental energy. I hope you've pinpointed key areas to address and energy-promoting actions that resonate with you. Even a small change can lead to meaningful progress.

In the final chapter, you'll pull together your reflections from your journey through The Happy Menopause Energy Clinic and put these insights into action. It's time for you to craft your personal Energy Action Plan – a tailored strategy to support your wellbeing and help you thrive through menopause and beyond!

BRINGING IT ALL TOGETHER

DESIGN YOUR PERSONAL ENERGY ACTION PLAN

Congratulations! You've made it all the way through The Happy Menopause Energy Clinic. As you worked through each section, you will have collected a series of action points that you've identified as relevant to you. In this section, you'll be bringing them together to create your own personal Energy Action Plan.

Throughout this guide, we've explored key themes that influence your energy levels. From the biochemistry of energy and the role of mitochondria to balancing nutrients and lifestyle choices, each step in your journey through The Happy Menopause Energy Clinic has provided insights and practical advice. Here's a quick recap of what you've covered so far:

- **Step 1:** The biochemistry of energy and the crucial role of the mitochondria. You've learned about the different ways that your diet and lifestyle can influence the action of mitochondria, both positively and negatively. You've also understood the impact of menopause on your energy levels.

- **Step 2:** The importance of keeping up to date with your health checks, so that you can take preventative measures to manage any underlying issues that might contribute to your lack of energy.
- **Step 3:** How to balance your macronutrients to support your physical and mental energy. Your 14-day Energy Boost Programme will have shown you just what a difference this can make to your vitality, mental clarity and productiveness.
- **Step 4:** The different micronutrient or functional imbalances that can impair your energy levels. You will have noted which ones are relevant to you, as well as strategies to address the issues.
- **Step 5:** The role of lifestyle choices in helping or hindering your energy levels, along with practical advice on areas you can work on.

The energy jigsaw

Achieving optimal energy is just like completing a jigsaw puzzle: each piece has its place. If even one piece is missing, the picture remains incomplete, disrupting the balance of your physical and mental energy. The themes we've explored – nutrition, lifestyle, health checks and more – are all interconnected. Think of them as the individual pieces of your energy puzzle. When they work together harmoniously, they sustain the energy you need to thrive in daily life.

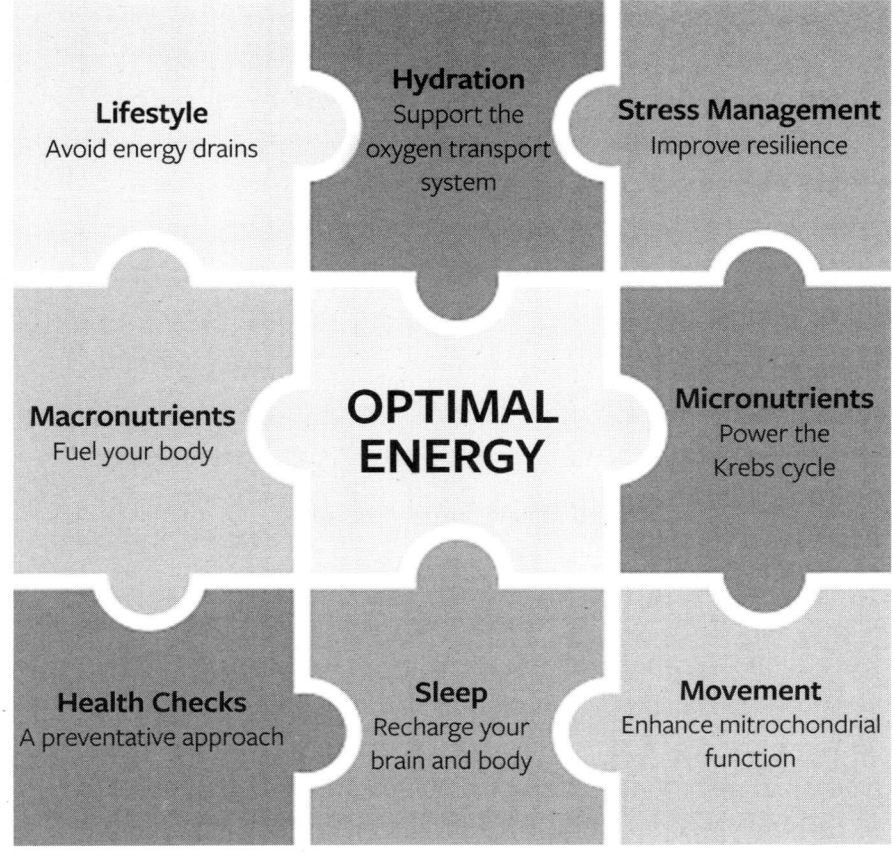

Lifestyle
Avoid energy drains

Hydration
Support the oxygen transport system

Stress Management
Improve resilience

Macronutrients
Fuel your body

OPTIMAL ENERGY

Micronutrients
Power the Krebs cycle

Health Checks
A preventative approach

Sleep
Recharge your brain and body

Movement
Enhance mitochondrial function

CREATE YOUR ENERGY ACTION PLAN

Now it's time to pull together a personalized energy action plan. Get your notebook out again, because you'll be integrating the SMART objectives you created in each reflection section to create a unified energy strategy that's just right for you.

1. **Gather your reflections and SMART objectives:** Read through your notes from each step and collate them in one place.
2. **Assess and prioritize:** You may have noted down a lot of different thoughts, which can feel overwhelming. Prioritize to avoid overload.
3. **Be systematic:** Work through your notes step by step, grouping similar ideas together.
4. **Identify themes:** Use a tally system to note recurring issues. Repetition often helps to highlight areas to tackle first.
5. **Colour-code your priorities:** Highlighting key points can help you navigate your plan more easily.
6. **Create a timeline:** Once you know what you want to achieve, build a practical, achievable schedule to get started.

Here are some examples of how you can structure your Energy Action Plan, as you work through your findings from each step:

Know Your Numbers: The Essential Health Checks Every Woman Needs (Step 2 Action Points)

Are you up to date with your health checks? Do you know what your latest test results are and what action might be required? Consider creating a table to track your progress. For example:

Health check	Last done	Action plan
Blood test	DD/MM/YYYY	Schedule follow-up appointment.
Blood pressure	DD/MM/YYYY	Review diet & lifestyle.

Nutrition Essentials – Complete the 14-Day Energy Boost Programme (Step 3 Action Points)

What did you learn from the 14-day Energy Boost Programme? Which macronutrients need your attention? Do you need to focus on hydration? Consider creating a table of action points; I've included a couple of examples to get you started.

Goal	Action plan
Increase protein	Add nuts & seeds to breakfast.
Stay hydrated	Drink a glass of water before meals.

Discover Targeted Solutions for Micronutrient Imbalances (Step 4 Action Points)

Use your energy quizzes to identify recurring issues. If necessary, revisit relevant sections for deeper insights. Tally recurring themes, such as nutrient deficiencies, and prioritize them, using these examples as a guide:

Nutrient	Key role	Action plan
Magnesium	Energy metabolism	Eat dark green leafy veg every day.
Vitamin B12	Red blood cell production	Book a blood test with the doctor.

Energy Drain or Energy Gain? Make Lifestyle Choices to Improve Your Vitality (Step 5 Action Points)

What lifestyle factors stood out? Use Step 5 to identify areas that need immediate attention. For example:

Issue	Action plan
Poor sleep	Set a bedtime wind-down routine.
Stress management	Take a red pen to my diary.

Bring it all together

Now it's time to bring everything together. Start by selecting five key objectives, so that you don't overload yourself. You can always build on this foundation later, adding new objectives as these changes become second nature and your confidence grows.

Identify one objective and create one action point for each of the B's: Balance, Boost, Boost, Banish and Behaviour. I suggest boosting one macronutrient and one micronutrient. However, if you feel the 14-Day Energy Boost Programme has already corrected the macronutrient balance, you may find it more beneficial to focus on two micronutrients instead.

BALANCE: Where do you need to find balance? Blood sugar imbalances are common, but perhaps another area stood out to you as needing attention.

BOOST: Which macronutrient do you need to increase? Are you lacking protein in your diet, are you overly restrictive with fat or have you cut out carbs completely?

BOOST: Is there a micronutrient that requires your focus? Do you need a blood test to check your levels? What dietary or supplement changes will help you improve this?

BANISH: What should you reduce or eliminate? Are you consuming too much caffeine or alcohol? Has excess sugar crept into your routine?

BEHAVIOUR: Which habits are hindering your progress? Do you need to improve your sleep hygiene? Should exercise become a priority? How can you reduce stress in your life?

Here's an example:

What	How	Action
BALANCE	Blood sugar	Swap to complex carbohydrate and avoid sugary foods.
BOOST	Protein	Eat protein with every meal, including one complete protein every day.
BOOST	Vitamin D	Take 1,000IU of vitamin D3 daily.
BANISH	Alcohol	Have at least four consecutive alcohol-free days each week.
BEHAVIOUR	Prioritize sleep	Set a digital-free hour before bed. Ban the phone from the bedroom.

Create a timeline

Turning objectives into actionable steps is key. Here's an example timeline:

Week 1	Week 2	Month 1	Month 2
Add a portion of dark green leafy vegetables (DGLV) to lunch.	Add another portion of DGLV to dinner.	Experiment with different types of DGLV to add variety, e.g. Swiss chard or cavolo nero.	Adjust your approach based on progress and results.

Remember, flexibility is key. Life can get in the way sometimes and unexpected challenges will crop up. That's perfectly okay. If need be, adapt your plan, reassess the timeline and keep moving forward. A thoughtful, measured approach is essential to long-term success as you build and refine your Energy Action Plan.

OVER TO YOU!

Well done on reaching the end of *The Happy Menopause Guide to Energy*! You've taken an important step toward boosting your energy and creating a healthier, more vibrant you. Now it's time to turn what you've learned into action – your brain and body will thank you for it.

Progress doesn't happen overnight. It's the small, consistent steps that lead to meaningful change. Start with something manageable – whether that's adding an extra portion of veg to your meals, eating more protein, taking a brisk walk or setting a regular bedtime.

Your journey to better energy starts now. Each step you take – no matter how small – brings you closer to the vibrant, balanced life you deserve. You're in control and the future is bright. Go for it!

APPENDIX

THE ENERGY PRODUCTION CHAIN REACTION

If you were intrigued by the simple explanation of energy production in Step 1 (see page 18), here's a closer look at the specifics of the chain reaction, so you can see exactly how the body does it.

The role of nutrition is key because the body takes the food we eat and combines it with oxygen to produce ATP (adenosine triphosphate) energy storage units in each cell. ATP is the body's energy currency, fuelling everything from muscle contraction to brain function.

This is how it works in simple terms:

1. **Fuel**

   When we eat carbohydrates, fats and proteins, they are broken down into smaller molecules. Carbohydrates become glucose, fats become fatty acids, and proteins become amino acids.

2. **Respiration**

Our body cells contain tiny structures called mitochondria, which act as energy power plants. Inside them, a process called respiration takes place. This is a sequence of reactions in which the food we've eaten reacts with oxygen and is converted into ATP energy molecules.

3. **ATP**

ATP molecules act like rechargeable batteries, storing and delivering energy when needed. They power everything from muscle movement to nerve signal transmission in the brain.

The chain reaction that leads to the creation of ATP is a multi-step process, with each phase playing a vital role. Micronutrients, such as vitamins and minerals, act as essential co-factors (catalyst molecules) that help enzymes facilitate each step of the energy production process.

BREAKING IT DOWN

Glycolysis

This phase takes place in the cell's cytoplasm, outside the mitochondria. Glycolysis is an anaerobic process, meaning it does not require oxygen. A glucose molecule is broken down into two molecules of pyruvate, producing a net gain of 2 ATP molecules.

During this process, high-energy electrons are transferred to a carrier molecule called NAD^+ (nicotinamide adenine dinucleotide), converting it into NADH. NADH acts as an electron shuttle, carrying these high-energy electrons to the next stages of energy production.

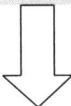

Citric acid cycle (Krebs cycle)

This phase occurs inside the mitochondria. In the citric acid cycle, pyruvate is further broken down into carbon dioxide, generating 2 ATP and transferring high-energy electrons to NAD^+ and another carrier molecule called FAD (flavin adenine dinucleotide), forming NADH and $FADH_2$. These electron carriers then move on to the next stage – the electron transport chain – where oxygen plays a key role in producing the majority of ATP.

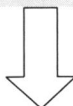

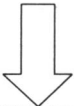

Electron transport chain (ETC)

This is the most energy-productive phase and takes place in the inner membrane of the mitochondria. Electrons from **NADH** and **FADH₂** are passed through a series of reactions involving oxygen, ultimately generating about **34 ATP** molecules in a process called **oxidative phosphorylation**. Oxygen acts as the final electron acceptor, forming water as a by-product.

Total ATP production

When you add up the ATP produced from all these stages, the total ATP yield per molecule of glucose is approximately:

- **2 ATP** from glycolysis
- **2 ATP** from the citric acid (Krebs cycle)
- **34 ATP** from the electron transport chain (ETC)
  Total = 38 ATP molecules per glucose molecule

The body continuously produces billions of ATP molecules every second, fuelling everything from basic bodily functions to intense physical activity and cognitive processes.

RESOURCES

Over the years, I've developed a range of menopause resources to support you. Start here for my menopause nutrition clinic, social media and The Happy Menopause collection:

🌐 Jackie's Nutrition Clinic: www.well-well-well.co.uk
📖 *The Happy Menopause: Smart Nutrition to Help You Flourish* (Watkins, 2020), by Jackie Lynch
🌐 The Happy Menopause Club: www.thehappymenopause.com
🎙 The Happy Menopause Podcast
📱 @wellwellwelluk

OTHER RESOURCES

These are some of my favourite books, websites and other resources, which I think you'll find really useful – and hopefully interesting too! I've handpicked them for you because they're just too good not to share. I hope they make your menopause journey a little easier and more empowering.

🌐 Menopause information websites & communities

The British Menopause Society (BMS): www.thebms.org.uk
The International Menopause Society: www.imsociety.org

The Menopause Society (North America): www.menopause.org
Henpicked: www.henpicked.net
Latte Lounge: www.lattelounge.co.uk
Menopause Matters: www.menopausematters.co.uk
Positive Pause: www.positivepause.co.uk
Women's Health Concern: www.womens-health-concern.org

⊕ Lifestyle websites

Amanda Thebe: www.amandathebe.com
Drink Less, Live Better: www.drinklesslivebetter.com
Max Richter Sleep: www.maxrichter-sleep.com
Pilates at Your Desk: www.pilatesatyourdesk.com
Yoga With Adriene: www.yogawithadriene.com

⚲ Podcasts

The Menopause Matters: Let's Talk
Magnificent Midlife
Menopause Whilst Black
Midlife Conversations
Postcards From Midlife
With All Due Respect

⊙ Instagram

@amanada.thebe
@jomoseley
@libbystevenson.wellbeing
@menohealthuk
@pilatesatyourdesk
@sampalmermidlifemakeover
@tanyadalton

⊕ Apps

The 7-Minute Work Out

Cara Fitness

Couch to 5k

Drink Awareness

Headspace

Squeezy

Zen Me

📖 Books

52 Ways to Walk: The Surprising Science of Walking for Wellness & Joy, One Week at a Time (Bloomsbury, 2022), by Annabel Streets

The Age Well Project: Easy Ways to Live a Longer, Healthier, Happier Life (Piatkus, 2019), by Annabel Streets & Susan Saunders

Beating Brain Fog: Your 30 Day Plan to Think Faster, Sharper, Better (Orion Spring, 2021), by Dr Sabina Brennan

Cracking the Menopause While Keeping Yourself Together (Bluebird, 2021), by Mariella Frostrup & Alice Smellie

The Expectation Effect: How Your Mindset Can Transform Your Life (Canongate, 2022), by David Robson

FAQs on Menopause (Sheldon Press, 2023), by Julie Robinson

Life Time: The New Science of the Body Clock, and How It Can Revolutionize Your Sleep and Health (Penguin, 2022), by Professor Russell Foster

Men ... Let's Talk Menopause: What's Going On and What You Can Do About It (Practical Inspiration Publishing, 2019), by Ruth Devlin

The Menopause Brain: The New Science Empowering Women to Navigate Midlife with Knowledge and Confidence (Allen & Unwin, 2024), by Dr Lisa Mosconi

Midlife Matters: Feel Empowered and Confident Every Step of the Way (DK Red, 2025), by Katie Taylor

The Super-Helper Syndrome: A Survival Guide for Compassionate People (Flint, 2024), by Jess Baker & Rod Vincent

Retirement Rebel: One Woman, One Motorhome, One Great Big Adventure (Vertebrate, 2022), by Siobhan Daniels

ABOUT THE AUTHOR

Jackie Lynch is an award-winning nutritionist, author, speaker and the founder of the WellWellWell nutrition clinic, where she has helped thousands of women take control of their health and navigate the menopause with confidence. Jackie originally studied languages and lived and worked in France for 13 years, where her deep interest in food and nutrition was influenced by the rich culinary culture there.

Now based in the UK, it was when she turned 40 that Jackie made a major career shift from a corporate job to pursue her passion for nutrition, embarking on a four-year course of study in nutritional therapy. This transformation not only reshaped her career but also inspired her to open her own clinic.

Passionate about breaking the taboo around menopause, she hosts the hugely popular The Happy Menopause podcast, which was shortlisted for the International Women's Podcast Awards in 2021, 2022, and 2024. She's also the founder of The Happy Menopause Club, a premium membership site offering expert nutrition resources and support for midlife women.

Jackie is the author of the bestselling *The Happy Menopause: Smart Nutrition to Help You Flourish* (Watkins, 2020), which was Highly Commended in the 2021 Health & Wellbeing Awards, and of *Va Va Voom:*

The 10-Day Energy Diet (Headline, 2017) and *The Right Bite: Smart Food Choices for Eating on the Go* (Nourish, 2016).

She regularly shares her expertise in national media and has appeared as a guest expert on radio and TV, including Channel 4's *Superfoods*. Her WellWellWell clinic was named Menopause Nutrition Clinic of the Year in the 2021 and 2022 London & South-East Prestige Awards.

A highly respected voice in the field, Jackie is a Fellow of the British Association for Nutrition & Lifestyle Medicine and a Member of the British Menopause Society. She also served as Chair of the Institute for Optimum Nutrition from 2011 to 2022.

Follow Jackie on social media at @WellWellWellUK or visit her website: www.well-well-well.co.uk

ACKNOWLEDGEMENTS

First and foremost, a heartfelt thank you to my editor, Fiona Robertson, for your unwavering belief in *The Happy Menopause* brand and its role in supporting women in midlife. It's been a pleasure working with you on this new addition to the collection, and I'm so very proud of the result!

I'm also extremely grateful to my agent, Barbara Levy, who is always quietly supportive in the background and ever ready to kick ideas around and to help me hone each new proposition.

To my brilliant family and friends, who are my constant cheerleaders and who kindly put up with my frequent complaints about how much work it is to write a book and how fiddly and painful the editorial process can be. Every time I embark on a new book, I blithely forget the challenges until it's too late, and every time, you kindly refrain from being anything other than utterly sympathetic and supportive! Thank you for the endless patience, the encouraging chats and messages, and for finding ways to tempt me away from my desk when I need a break – I couldn't do it without you.

To my colleagues and peers both in the field of nutrition and in the wider world of women's health, thank you for your collaboration, insight and dedication to empowering women to take charge of their health. Your knowledge and expertise continually inspire me to deepen my own understanding of the powerful connection between diet, lifestyle and the menopause.

A sincere thank you to the whole team behind this book – from the editorial team who guided me through the whole process and ensured that every word was carefully considered, to the designers who brought the pages to life with their inspired approach, the marketing team who have so brilliantly spread the word and the sales team who are sending it on its way into the world. Your expertise and hard work have helped turn this vision into a reality that can make a tangible difference to women in midlife.

Finally, to every woman reading this book – thank you for trusting me to guide you on this transformative journey. Your health matters, and I hope the insights shared within these pages will help you feel revitalized, empowered and inspired to live your best life.

With gratitude,

Jackie

INDEX

Note: page numbers in **bold** refer to diagrams.